Contents

THE LEARNING CENTRE
HAM...
LC...
G...
LONDON W14 9BL
0181 741 1688

KU-163-777

Appraising *Your* Staff

SECOND EDITION

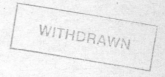

PHILIP MOON

THE LEARNING CENTRE
HAMMERSMITH AND WEST
LONDON COLLEGE
GLIDDON ROAD
LONDON W14 9BL
0181 741 1688

HAMMERSMITH AND WEST LONDON COLLEGE

293998

YOURS TO HAVE AND TO HOLD

BUT NOT TO COPY

The publication you are reading is protected by copyright law. This means that the publisher could take you and your employer to court and claim heavy legal damages if you make unauthorised photocopies from these pages. Photocopying copyright material without permission is no different from stealing a magazine from a newsagent, only it doesn't seem like theft.

The Copyright Licensing Agency (CLA) is an organisation which issues licences to bring photocopying within the law. It has designed licensing services to cover all kinds of special needs in business, education and government.

If you take photocopies from books, magazines and periodicals at work your employer should be licensed with CLA. Make sure you are protected by a photocopying licence.

The Copyright Licensing Agency Limited, 90 Tottenham Court Road, London, W1P 0LP. Tel: 0171 436 5931. Fax: 0171 436 3986.

First published in 1993
This edition published in 1997

Apart from any fair dealing for the purposes of research or private study, or criticism or review, as permitted under the Copyright, Designs and Patents Act 1988, this publication may only be reproduced, stored or transmitted, in any form or by any means, with the prior permission in writing of the publishers, or in the case of reprographic reproduction in accordance with the terms and licences issued by the CLA. Enquiries concerning reproduction outside those terms should be sent to the publishers at the undermentioned address:

Kogan Page Limited
120 Pentonville Road
London N1 9JN

© Philip Moon 1993, 1997

The right of Philip Moon to be identified as author of this work has been asserted by him in accordance with the Copyright, Designs and Patents Act 1988.

HAMMERSMITH AND WEST
LONDON COLLEGE
LEARNING CENTRE
Business Studies

14 AUG 1998

DAW B563503 £10.99

293998

658.3125

British Library Cataloguing in Publication Data
A CIP record for this book is available from the British Library.

ISBN 0 7494 2454 0

Typeset by Saxon Graphics Ltd, Derby
Printed in England by Clays Ltd, St Ives plc

1 *Introduction*

The purpose of this book is to help you, as a manager, develop the understanding and skills you need to get the best out of staff appraisal in the interest of yourself, your staff and your organisation.

The book assumes that your organisation already operates an appraisal scheme. It should also be of interest if, either from a line-management or personnel perspective, you want to explore the implications of introducing or reforming appraisal. You will see that I have included in this revised edition an appendix on 'Implementing an appraisal system'. Although not its explicit intention, the book should also be useful to appraisees in helping them to get the best from appraisal. You may, of course, be wearing two hats as both appraiser and appraisee, or even three as appraiser, appraisee and personnel specialist.

Effective staff appraisal isn't simply a matter of 'going through the motions': holding ritualistic interviews and mechanically completing forms at the behest of the personnel department, before returning to the 'more important' tasks of day-to-day management. On the contrary, appraisal is a tool to help managers manage. You should undertake it not just with the requirements of the system in mind but more importantly, with the needs and interests of your own staff uppermost. Whatever appraisal system you're working with, whatever its constraints and whatever your obligations under it, make it work for you and your staff. Often this will mean 'going the extra mile'.

To meet this responsibility you need to develop your understanding of your own organisation's appraisal system. The examination of appraisal systems which this book presents should assist this process by providing you with a context in which to assess your own particular system. This should help you clarify your understanding of its main features, its objectives and its strengths and weaknesses. Appreciating the weaknesses of your system (and it's unlikely that your system doesn't have any) can be extremely valuable in helping you to avoid some of the pitfalls of appraisal.

As well as understanding systems, the effective appraiser also needs to understand people and what makes them tick. This is particularly so as part of your objective in appraising staff is to help them improve performance. This book will provide you with an examination of the way motivational factors impact upon staff performance and help you develop practical strategies for dealing with individual members of staff. It should, however, be emphasised that managing people is not a matter of applying simplistic standardised formulae. People management is an art. It requires subtlety and flexibility.

On the skills side, getting the best from appraisal involves developing and honing a range of techniques. These include the skill of identifying training and development needs as well as the multi-faceted skills of leading appraisal discussions. Many of the skills involved are those which managers use every day – communicating, listening, questioning and criticising. These skills are acquired through life and work experience, but this book should help you refine these skills and ensure that you adopt a planned and structured approach to appraisal. Even if much of this approach is common sense, common sense is, alas, not always common practice!

A few words on terminology

Many organisations avoid the word 'appraisal' and choose different terminology for carefully considered reasons. The very word 'appraisal' is sometimes seen as having negative connotations. Thus there are a variety of terms in use such as 'staff development review' or 'performance review' or even 'development needs assessment'. The particular terminology adopted may reflect a particular emphasis of a particular system. This book uses the term 'appraisal' in a generic sense to cover a wide range of systems. Here 'appraisal' is simply defined as 'a formal documented system for the periodic review of an individual's performance'.

This definition focuses on what may be considered the

essential or defining ingredients of appraisal. The formality and documentation are essential elements as they distinguish 'appraisal' from the day-to-day feedback an individual may receive from his/her boss on an informal and oral basis. The point that appraisal is periodic, distinguishes it from the kind of formal review which might take place as the result of specific circumstances, such as consideration for promotion, disciplinary situations or the completion of a probationary period.

You might also note that this definition does not refer to an 'interview' – some appraisal systems operate without an interview being a necessary or obligatory part of the process. Nor indeed does this definition talk of objective setting, training needs assessment, promotion and career prospect reviews. These may be encompassed within an appraisal but they are by no means common to all systems and should not be regarded as defining characteristics.

The point is simply this. This book takes a broad definition of appraisal so that, whatever the name, scope or style of the system you operate, it can help you operate it more effectively to everyone's advantage.

You might also like to think about other terminology associated with appraisal. While throughout this book I've used the words 'appraiser' and 'appraisee', some organisations (particularly if they are avoiding the word 'appraisal') prefer to use the words 'manager' and 'job-holder' or 'reviewer' and 'reviewee'. Another choice to consider is whether to refer to the appraisal 'interview' or the appraisal 'discussion'. The first edition of this book used the word 'interview' throughout. For this updated edition, I've preferred the word 'discussion'. 'Interview' has the sense of something which is done _to_ someone, whereas 'discussion' suggests greater mutuality and something which is done _with_ someone. When talking with colleagues, and particularly with staff, it's probably helpful if you use the words consistent with your organisation's scheme.

Note. The book is written on the assumption that as appraiser you are your appraisees' direct line manager or immediate boss. This is the way most, but not all, appraisal systems work. If you are appraising staff who do not report directly to you, the book will still be relevant to your needs. You will need to place particular emphasis on gathering information from whomever appraisees report to and, of course, your strategies for helping appraisees improve performance will have to involve their immediate supervisors. Even when the appraiser is intended to be the line manager, some organisations are rather loose or vague in their reporting structures. If you've got to manage under a new system make sure you know who your appraisees are going to be.

Dimensions of appraisal design

Each appraisal scheme will have its particular combination of features which contribute to its uniqueness. Here are some of the design dimensions which will vary from scheme to scheme.

- Who appraises – line manager, two-up manager, or 'mentor'?
- How often and when – annually, six-monthly, staggered or concentrated?
- Scale markings or narrative report?
- Overall assessment or no overall assessment?
- Review of 'inputs' or of 'outcomes' and objectives?

---

2 Why appraise?

Over the last 15 years, more and more organisations have introduced some form of appraisal system. While appraisal may have its problems, and it is certainly arguable that it is not successful or appropriate in all situations, this growing use of appraisal suggests that many organisations find it a worthwhile process. Operating an appraisal system requires quite an investment of resources by the organisation and time and effort by the appraising manager. These investments need to be justified in terms of the benefits which ensue.

In this chapter we examine these benefits and the reasons for adopting and operating an appraisal system – why, in theory at least, appraisal is seen as a 'good thing'. In Chapter 3 we'll have a look at some of the problems appraisal faces and why it's not always seen by everyone as being such a good thing in practice.

The specific benefits of any appraisal system will depend upon the objectives it is intended to achieve and the extent to which the system is designed and operated to meet those objectives. Although not all the benefits considered below are mutually compatible, it is possible to talk at a general level about the potential benefits which appraisal can bring.

I would suggest that these benefits can be classified under three headings:

- the benefits to the appraisee;
- the benefits to the appraiser; and
- the benefits for the organisation.

Clearly there will be an overlap between the three. After all, anything which benefits the individual employee should also benefit both his/her appraising manager and the organisation as a whole. As an appraising manager yourself, you will be concerned not only for your own interests, but also for those of your staff and the organisation which employs you.

Because the philosophy of this book is that appraisal is something which is done *for* staff, it makes sense to begin our review of benefits from the appraisee's perspective.

Benefits to the appraisee

Receiving feedback

The first and perhaps most obvious benefit to the individual is the opportunity to receive feedback on his/her performance. Everyone needs feedback. They need to know how well they are doing, or if what they are doing is not right. Without feedback individuals can feel vulnerable. 'Is my work really valued?' 'What does the boss *really* think of me?'

It might be argued that a good boss provides feedback on a day-to-day basis. This is, of course, true. But such feedback tends to be unstructured and *ad hoc*. It tends also to relate to specific tasks in hand. Appraisal provides the individual with the opportunity to have his/her job and performance looked at as a whole, in a balanced and thought-through way. It offers an occasion to have achievements formally recognised and documented, and the chance to bring certain achievements to the boss's notice which might otherwise have been overlooked. (Professional development)

The fact that this feedback is documented also provides the appraisee with a certain amount of protection. After all, if there is a written record showing that the appraisee is doing a good job, his/her boss can hardly turn round shortly afterwards and say: 'Your performance isn't up to scratch ...!'

It also needs to be recognised that, where there is no appraisal system, it does not mean that individual employees are not being appraised. It merely means that appraisal is taking place in an unstructured way, behind closed doors, without the individual knowing how he/she is being assessed, and without him/her having the opportunity to partake actively in the process.

Opportunity to feed back to boss

Appraisees' performances are affected not only by their own strengths and weaknesses, but also by the way they are man-

aged. As an appraisee's line manager, you may (albeit unwittingly) be acting as a block to his/her effective performance.
  The appraisee may feel that:

- you don't give him/her enough attention;
- you don't understand some of the particular problems involved in the job;
- you haven't provided (or fought hard enough for) the necessary resources – material, human, or whatever;
- you don't give him/her enough authority;
- you are interrupting constantly;
- you don't explain clearly enough what you want;
- you're too willing to commit the department to do things it's not able to do.

Opportunities to discuss such issues can be highly valued by appraisees: not merely as a means of resolving specific problems, but also because they provide them with a sense of participating in their own management.

  Of course it might be argued that in a good working relationship, staff will feel free to provide such feedback to their bosses anyway. It's quite typical for managers to say: 'If anyone's ever got any problems or suggestions, they know they can always bring them to me. I'm always available to my staff.' However, many bosses are not as accessible or responsive as they perceive themselves to be. The fact that appraisal is a formal system, provides staff with a little 'protection' to say things that they might not have been happy to say otherwise. Often this means that they can feed back to their boss in a more candid way than they would feel free to do during the course of a day-to-day conversation.

Having training needs identified

Appraisal provides an opportunity to have personal training needs examined, so that appraisers can develop their skills, perform more efficiently and gain the benefits of doing a better job. If you don't provide individuals with the opportunity to have their training needs formally assessed, they may feel that the organisation has no real commitment to, or interest in, them. This in turn can result in demotivation and a lack of commitment to the job.

Opportunity to discuss career prospects and promotion

Understandably many people are concerned about their future. 'Am I likely to be in line for promotion?' 'What are the long-term prospects for me with this organisation?' These are issues which you need to discuss with your staff and appraisal can provide an opportunity for an individual to receive a frank assessment of his/her prospects. If the organisation has a formal system for recommending people for promotion (such as a promotion board), then individuals need to be told whether they are considered ready for promotion or not. If they are not considered ready for promotion, they have a right to know why not, and to discuss with you what action they need to take to make themselves more promotable.

A discussion of promotional prospects is not always part and parcel of an appraisal system. Many organisations establish separate systems for career counselling, recognising that discussing prospects during appraisal may blur the focus on current performance. Nonetheless the point here is that many individuals do need to discuss their careers and that appraisal can provide an opportunity which might not otherwise be available.

Clarifying objectives, job descriptions and priorities

A formal appraisal provides your staff with the opportunity to discuss the objectives of their jobs with you. It's surprising how often people are unclear as to what these are. The result is that they find it very difficult to set priorities and determine those tasks that are truly important to their role in the team and the organisation. It's not uncommon for a member of staff to have a view of their job that differs from the boss's. For instance, they might concentrate on some aspect of the job which was given particular emphasis during their original selection interview yet which was never intended to be the most important part of the job.

Clearly, if people are to perform well in their jobs, they need to know what it is they're supposed to achieve and also what the criteria of effective performance are. Appraisal can help to iron out the ambiguities.

Discussion of job design chopT - 5/6

Appraisal also provides an opportunity to consider issues of job design. Is the job varied and interesting? Does it utilise the full talents of the appraisee? Could he/she take on more responsibility? Could important aspects of the job be done in a different way? Is the job too demanding – could certain elements of it be dropped, or is there a need to bring in extra resources?

Appraisal thus provides staff with the chance to suggest ways in which their jobs could be made more fulfilling, efficient, or easier. These are important aspects of motivation and job satisfaction which will be further examined in Chapters 5 and 6.

Benefits of performance-related pay (PRP)

Performance-related pay can be a contentious issue and if your organisation operates a performance-related pay system, you need to be aware of some of the problems this may cause for the appraisal process. These are examined in the next chapter. However, as well as involving difficulties, performance-related pay also provides benefits and opportunities for the individual. After all, performance-related pay allows good performers to receive material recognition for their good performance. It follows that some system of appraisal is necessary if individuals are to be assessed for such rewards and if they are to be told what they need to do to improve performance to the level which will trigger a higher award the next time round.

Benefits to the line manager

We have already noted that as a line manager you will gain from any benefits your staff derive from an appraisal system. If the aim of appraisal is to improve the performance of staff and if this is achieved, then clearly appraisal will have helped you to meet your objective of making the best use of the human resources for which you are responsible.

Ch. 13   *see involvement of staff*

Feedback to appraisee

Appraisal provides you with a formal and structured opportunity to feed back information to your staff. It allows you to show that you've noticed what has been done well. It also allows you to tackle any problems or any criticisms you may have. Given the formality of the process, you may feel able to tackle contentious issues (which might otherwise be swept under the carpet) and any criticisms you make will be within the context of the appraisee's good performance in other parts of the job.

The appraisal should not be regarded as the sole opportunity to express your criticisms and it's wrong to store them up for annual 'blood letting'. Nonetheless, there may be 'downsides' to an individual's performance for which the appraisal provides the appropriate discussion forum. Without a formal system there is a possibility that particularly difficult issues may be ignored. Chapter 13 discusses the skills of constructive criticism.

Setting and clarifying objectives

In our earlier discussion of benefits to the appraisee, we saw that many people are unclear about the objectives of their job. It is important for you to clarify these objectives with staff so that they can set the right priorities and give their time to the right sort of work, ensuring that efforts are directed towards achieving your departmental goals and the goals of the organisation.

Appraisal also allows you to look forward and to plan work for the next period – setting (or agreeing) objectives and targets which are achievable and motivating, and integrated with those of the department and organisation.

Identification of training needs *Ch. 8*

Appraisal provides an opportunity for a structured analysis of the individual's training needs and a forum for a two-way discussion, providing you with the opportunity to air your own ideas and gather those of the appraisee.

Training is not, however, the solution to all performance problems, nor is it intended to be a reward for good performance. (The processes of identifying and meeting training needs are discussed in further detail in Chapter 8.)

Audit of team's strengths and weaknesses

Appraisal allows you to take stock of the skills and talents, strengths and weaknesses of your team. This should help you make more effective use of team members. It may help you to realise that the team has underexploited strengths which could enable you to offer a new, additional, or better service to the organisation or the customer. For instance, if you run a clerical support unit you may discover that one of your staff has the aptitudes and experience to enable your department to offer an in-house design facility.

On the other hand, appraisal may help you to recognise that you don't have the personnel to meet the department's remit. It should thus help you to decide what skills are needed and what type of people you should recruit to complement your current team. More radically, you might even decide that some of your departmental objectives are unrealistic given the human resource base available. Consequently objectives may need to be redrawn to make the most of the resources you actually have at your disposal.

Receiving feedback on own management style

We've already suggested that many people welcome the opportunity to feed back to their bosses their views about how they are being managed. This process (although possibly painful) can be extremely valuable for you as a manager. If the way you manage somebody affects their performance, you should be able to do something to improve the situation and help them to work more effectively. Although many managers regard themselves as approachable and responsive to criticism, individual employees may need to be encouraged to provide the feedback that managers need. An appraisal system can provide the necessary opportunity and help your staff to clarify and articulate their view of your management style.

Exploring and resolving problems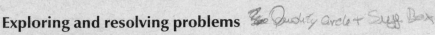

The exploration and resolution of problems may be seen as part of the feedback process. However, all problems require a two-way discussion and commitment by all parties concerned to the action necessary to resolve them. Appraisal can provide you with the opportunity to talk through such problems and agree action accordingly. (It is important, however, to be sure to appraise *all* aspects of performance and not to allow the appraisal process to become hijacked by one or two thorny issues.)

Reducing staff turnover

High levels of staff turnover can be extremely costly. They cause disruption and represent a loss of skills and experience. New staff take time to be trained.

People leave for a variety of reasons. However, if appraisal provides a means for tackling the issues behind some of those reasons, then it can help to reduce turnover and its associated costs, and make your job easier and more effective.

Benefits to the organisation

Improved performance through commitment to staff

The organisation should benefit in the same ways as the line manager through having staff who perform better. A well-operated appraisal system can be taken as an indication of the organisation's commitment to the welfare, rights and interests of each individual employee.

A minimum standard of good management

The point has already been made that good managers will communicate regularly with their staff. However, not all managers are instinctively good managers. Many feel themselves to be under such time pressures that they don't give the time they should to their staff. An appraisal system enables the organisation to ensure that all managers do give at least some quality time and consideration to their staff. It reminds managers that staff management is a central responsibility of their jobs, and ensures that every individual gets at least some attention and formal feedback.

This is an important justification for operating an appraisal system. Getting the best out of people cannot simply be a matter of designing good management systems. Good management requires the individual manager to do more than merely meet the requirements of the system. As we've argued, you have to be prepared to 'go the extra mile' to make the system work effectively. Nonetheless, a good appraisal system at least establishes a minimum standard of management.

Aggregating training needs

Appraisal is often associated with the identification of training needs. One of the benefits to the organisation is that it allows individual needs to be aggregated to develop the organisation's training plan. If a particular training need is identified in several appraisals, there is a need, and opportunity, for the organisation to develop in-house courses or other means of dealing with it.

Manpower and succession planning

Appraisal allows the organisation to take a look at its staff resources as a whole. It provides a source of information which can answer questions such as:

- Have we got the right sort of people to match the needs of the organisation as it develops over the next five years?
- Do we have people whom we are going to be able to promote to fill the vacancies which will occur naturally?
- Are the individuals we identified as likely to succeed to higher posts, performing in line with our expectations and are they indeed suitable for such promotion?

Used appropriately, the appraisal system can help the personnel department to develop the human resources strategies needed to meet the medium- to long-term goals of the organisation.

Test of selection processes

One benefit which is often overlooked is the opportunity to assess the effectiveness of selection and recruitment methods. Every organisation needs to ask the key question: 'Are the people we have recruited performing as well as we expected them to?' If, in general, the answer to this question is 'no', then further questions should be asked about the recruitment and selection processes adopted by the organisation. These might include:

- Are we advertising in the right places?
- Do we need to adopt more stringent selection tests?
- Are we recruiting the right calibre of person?
- Do we need to offer more money?
- Do we need to review our induction programme?

Any changes in the recruitment process should also be monitored through the appraisal system.

- Has the introduction of psychometric testing led to our selecting staff who perform consistently better than those we selected previously?

The danger is that without an appraisal system some of these key personnel issues might be overlooked. Admittedly, however, it's better not to leave the validation of selection processes to appraisal. Ideally this should form part of a probationary review at the end of an initial (say) six-month period after appointment. Unfortunately, proper probationary reviews are more often a matter of the exception rather than the rule.

3 The problems with appraisal

While in the previous chapter we explored the potential benefits of appraisal, it is appropriate also to admit that appraisal has its problems. Indeed, many managers who believe that appraisal is a good thing in principle are often far less enthusiastic in practice. If you are to be an effective appraiser, it is as important to recognise the problems and pitfalls as it is to appreciate the benefits. It is certainly worth exploring any subconscious unease you may feel towards the appraisal process. The problems may lie with the system design, the expectations, attitudes and skills of the appraisers and appraisees, or even the culture and structure of the organisation. Exploring these problems and recognising the constraints should help you address the key question 'What do I need to do to make appraisal work more effectively?'

Understanding the problems

Some of the misgivings and problems commonly identified by appraising managers are examined below.

Appraisal takes too much time

Nearly all managers are busy and will complain that they are short of time. While sympathising with managers who face such pressures, it is important to recognise that this is an issue of priorities, not time. Complaining that there is inadequate time for effective appraisal reflects the attitude that appraisal is given a lower priority than other management responsibilities. Indeed, many managers fail to appreciate that the management of people is not just an administrative task bolted on to their jobs: it is actually a central part of their responsibility and requires an appropriate allocation of time.

If completing the forms, preparing for, and conducting the appraisal discussion takes you four hours per appraisee (and it might take more or less), those four hours represent a very small proportion of the total number of hours that particular individual works for you during the year as a whole – seven and a half hours a day for 220 days amounts to 1650 hours per year.

Having made this point, it is fair to say that appraisers can only be expected to give priority to appraisal if they believe the system delivers at least some of the benefits we noted in Chapter 2. In other words, appraisers won't feel happy about giving time to something they don't see as being worthwhile.

Complicated paperwork

Another complaint is that the documentation is complicated, cumbersome and/or facile. This may be a reasonable objection and there is an onus on the designers of systems to avoid these problems.

However, you should remember that the documentation is not the sole or even primary end. It's a mistake to think that all you need to do to satisfy the system is to complete the form as quickly as possible and send it back to the personnel department. Always remember that the primary objective is to carry out a structured review of performance and to have a meaningful discussion with each member of your team. The paperwork may provide the framework for that discussion, or it may merely act as the means by which the personnel department ensures that the process takes place.

Never seems to lead to anything

It's difficult for both appraisers and appraisees to feel enthusiastic about a process which never seems to deliver anything. 'Here we are again for our annual chat – time to go through the motions again.' As an appraiser it's essential for you to ensure that appraisal is action-orientated and that both you and the appraisee leave the discussion with clear and agreed action points for each to undertake.

Take a careful look at the documentation which accompanies your system and the requirement it makes for you to list action points. There is often a confusion here between two distinct types of action point. On the one hand, there are actions which are tasks and objectives set for the appraisee for the next period such as 'produce new product brochure'. On the other hand, there are actions which appraiser and appraisee agree to undertake to help the appraisee to perform better, such as identifying a training course, attending a particular meeting or acquiring additional resources.

Even if your formal documentation doesn't make this distinction, there's no reason why you and your appraisee should not make a separate record of action points. Indeed, I would regard a record of agreed action points as an essential outcome of any appraisal discussion. There's no difference here between an appraisal and other business meetings. The outcome of a well-conducted meeting should be a series of action points with each action point allocated to the appropriate party.

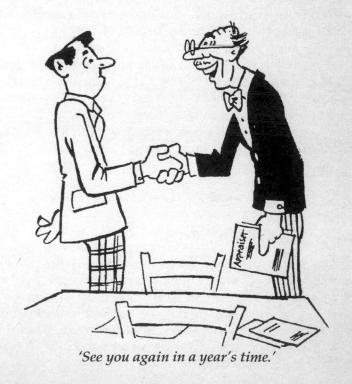

'See you again in a year's time.'

Monitoring the implementation of the action points on an ongoing basis is vital. The appraisal system will be brought into disrepute if the next time action points are reviewed is at an appraisal discussion one year later.

Only promise to do those things that you can do. Don't commit yourself to things you can't deliver. You may not be in a position to give someone their own secretary or a new office and you shouldn't promise to do so. You can, however, commit yourself to saying that you will take up the case and will let your appraisee know your boss's response.

Don't like playing 'God'

Many managers feel personally uneasy about sitting in judgement over their colleagues. This is particularly so if these judgements (which are ultimately subjective) directly affect the pay or promotional prospects of someone with whom they work closely. While this is understandable, you should remember that assessing staff performance is a part of your managerial responsibility. It's not an option. Assertiveness and the willingness to face up to difficulties are essential attributes of the effective appraiser.

Note, however, that your system may not require you to make an overall assessment of your appraisees – either in terms of rank, mark or comment. Many appraisal systems are concerned not so much with *assessing* performance as with *enhancing* performance.

Don't like criticising staff

The point was made in the last chapter that one of the benefits of appraisal was that it may make it easier to raise points of criticism. Nonetheless many appraisers still feel uncomfortable with the requirement to criticise staff which appraisal may impose. Criticising is a difficult business and many managers fear that if they handle it badly it will backfire.

The answer has to lie not in avoiding giving criticism but in developing criticising skills. These, as we have noted, are discussed in more detail in Chapter 13. At this stage, however, it may be helpful to anticipate one or two points of that discussion. First, as an appraiser you are looking at an individual's performance and the ways in which it can be enhanced. You're not criticising the person themselves: you're criticising their behaviour. Always be wary of making personal attacks. Second, the appraisal discussion should not be regarded as the occasion to offload criticisms which you have been storing up for a long time. Constructive criticism should be a normal part of the day-to-day transactions between a manager and his/her staff. This reinforces the point that to be a good appraiser you need to have good and open ongoing relations with your staff. Appraisal is not a substitute for good day-to-day management.

Arguments over pay

I've encountered several organisations where the relationship between appraisal and performance related pay was either ambiguous or poorly understood. Often the phrase 'performance-related pay' is used where the term 'discretionary pay element' might be more accurate. If you're to handle issues of pay effectively, it's important to have a clear understanding of the mechanisms through which your organisation makes discretionary pay awards.

Where pay is related to performance, appraisal can become a focus for arguments over pay. It can encourage appraisees to 'talk-up' their performance in the hope of receiving greater rewards and may inhibit frank discussion of problem areas. Don't let this happen. If your appraisal system puts you into a difficult position, adopt a damage limitation strategy. Focus discussion on how performance could be improved so as to allow the appraisee the opportunity of a greater reward next year.

Difficulty of assessing performance objectively

Whatever the system of appraisal, it is difficult to make objective assessments of performance. To an extent any assessment is bound to be subjective. You must, however, do your best to avoid bias and prejudice.

Negative appraisees

Even folks you get on well with on a day-to-day basis can turn difficult or 'bolshy' in the appraisal situation if you handle it badly. This may be partly to do with the appraisee's expectations of the system. Not unreasonably, appraisees may be sceptical – often they may be downright cynical. They may well suspect that a hidden agenda lies behind the process. Appraisees often feel that they are cast in a passive role in which they are to be the victims of the system. As a manager, you have an important role to play in helping your appraisees to understand the benefits of the system to them and the importance of their active participation in the process.

Making appraisal work

Identifying these problems helps us to focus on identifying what we need to make appraisal work. The main ingredients include some of the following features:

Committed appraisers who believe that appraisal is worthwhile and who have a willingness to invest appropriate time and effort.

Committed appraisees who believe, similarly, that appraisal is worthwhile and that there is something of real value in it for them.

Skilled appraisers who understand how the system operates and have the requisite skills both to analyse performance and to lead a constructive discussion.

Enlightened appraisees who know how the system operates, what's expected from them and who also come fully prepared to participate actively in their own performance review.

An appropriate system which has clear objectives and operates effectively to achieve those objectives without becoming bureaucratic and cumbersome and which ensures that documentation is user-friendly and that performance measures are realistic.

There are, of course, many other points which could be added, particularly appertaining to system design and operation. Some of these issues will be explored further in the next chapter. The important point to recognise at this stage is that appraisal can't be perfect, but that it's still worthwhile. Much of the responsibility for making it worthwhile lies with you as the appraiser. You have the responsibility to show commitment and to develop your own skills and understanding. You have the responsibility to create a positive attitude amongst your staff and to ensure that they understand the system and come properly prepared. You have the responsibility to make the system operate as well as it can. This may mean going beyond its basic requirements and using your discretion in line with the spirit of the system rather than necessarily adhering strictly to its letter.

Appraisal as a continuous process

One of the points which follows from this discussion and which needs to be emphasised is that appraisal should not be regarded as an annual, one-off exercise. The process needs to be a continuous one of monitoring performance and of providing regular feedback, advice and counselling. The formal appraisal system establishes a framework with its requirements for formal discussion and the completion of documentation, but 'making appraisal work' means working at it all year long. Again, this may mean going beyond the basic requirements of your formal system. It requires an attitude of mind which sees appraisal as a valuable tool in helping individual members of staff to perform effectively.

4 Which appraisal system?

Understanding the system

The purpose of this chapter is to help you develop your understanding of your own appraisal system. It attempts to do this by highlighting the contrast between the system you use and the systems operated by other organisations. The comparisons which you draw will help you to focus attention on some of the potential pitfalls in reviewing performance and completing your system's documentation.

The first, most obvious, point is that there is no one system which is 'right'. The system which is 'right' is the one which best fits the organisation, its culture, and its people. This principle of 'the best fit' is known as 'the contingency theory of management': the features of a system should be 'contingent' upon the circumstances, ie designed to meet the needs of the situation. The right appraisal system is also one which meets its own objectives. In other words, the right system is the one which delivers the outcomes the organisation has decided it wants from appraisal.

One of the critical factors in making your system work is that you should be thoroughly familiar with it, understand what it's trying to achieve and what (if anything) it's trying to measure. Often a problem occurs when appraisers think they understand their system when in fact they do not. This may be because superficially it resembles one with which they are familiar while it is actually rather different. Alternatively, it may be because the system has been gradually reformed with the result that it has actually changed significantly but subtly, so that the changes have not been consciously recognised by appraisers. Yet again, the confusion may result from ambiguities in the documentation which supports and explains the system. Often, possible differences of interpretation are never realised by the system's designers.

The range of systems

Appraisal systems come in many forms. Your own system may well be a blend of a number of different features intended to serve the various objectives your system may have.

Some systems place their emphasis on measuring performance in terms of strengths and weaknesses. (Though 'weaknesses' are sometimes euphemistically referred to as 'areas for improvement'.) Other systems are based primarily on a latter-day form of what was once called 'Management by Objectives' (MBO). This involves assessing performance against the objectives of the previous period and setting new ones for the next period. These two approaches can be contrasted, albeit crudely, as 'input' and 'output' systems. The 'strengths and weaknesses' approach looks at what the appraisee puts into the job (inputs), MBO looks at what's achieved in the job – the outputs. Both approaches have their value and elements of each may be combined in a single system. By itself each approach also has its limitations. The 'strengths and weaknesses' approach fails to place enough emphasis on the need to achieve. The MBO approach emphasises what's been achieved, not how it's been achieved and what more could be achieved. MBO may also fail to distinguish whether targets were achieved in spite of, rather than because of, the appraisee's contribution.

Systems differ also not only in what they measure, but also in how they measure. Some systems involve rating systems by which marks are given either for overall performance and/or for performance in specified areas. Some systems involve a ranking process in which members of staff are ranked in order of their performance. This may be tied into a performance-related pay system – the top 10 per cent of performers receiving one level of increase, the middle 80 per cent receiving another, and the bottom 10 per cent receiving another (or none at all). Some appraisal systems eschew marking scales altogether and rely instead on narrative comments. Usually this means writing comments under a number of headings, but some organisations simply use a blank piece of paper as their appraisal documentation, allowing appraisers to structure reports as they wish.

Some systems do not involve measuring performance at all – neither quantitatively nor qualitatively. These systems focus instead on identifying blockages to effective performance and job satisfaction and actions to deal with these blockages. Of course, this will involve an analytical review of past performance, but the appraisal documentation itself does not require the assessment of that past performance to be part of the appraisal record.

Examples of these different approaches and features are given below. Examining these examples should help you to focus on the requirements of your own system and identify any areas of ambiguity. Where you do uncover ambiguity, seek clarification from whoever it is who has the responsibility for managing your system.

Sample system 1

Sample 1 (see Figure 4.1) is an `input' type system. It also involves producing an overall ranking of performance within the department. In some ways its simplicity is very attractive (the documentation extends only to one side of A4 paper), but there are dangers. The appraiser only has a series of boxes to complete and there is a temptation to do this in a mechanical or ritualistic way. Space for comments is very limited and there is no place for a record of agreed action points. Unfortunately this kind of system can too easily be reduced to a quick form-filling exercise. If your system is like this, you need to go a lot further if you and your staff are really to gain the full benefits of appraisal.

Sample system 2

Sample 2 (see Figure 4.2) is a more sophisticated example of an 'input' system. Here one of the prime objectives is to produce an overall assessment by analysing a number of 'performance areas'. Though this is not a bad system, it includes ambiguities which lead many appraisers to operate it badly.

NAME	DATE	RANKING

PERFORMANCE ASSESSMENT

Use the following codes to indicate assessment of performance in each area.

ER = exceeded requirements   FM = fully met the requirements
SM = sometimes met the   NM = did not meet minimum
      requirements   requirements

TECHNOLOGY OF JOB	__	**ACHIEVEMENT OF RESULTS**	__
TECHNICAL KNOWLEDGE	__	QUALITATIVE	__
WORK ORG. & PRACTICALITY		QUANTITATIVE	__
(OWN JOB)	__	COST CONSCIOUSNESS	__
COMMUNICATION SKILLS	__		
SELF-MOTIVATION	__	**HUMAN RELATIONS**	__
INITIATIVE AND DRIVE	__	PEER RELATIONSHIP	
ACCEPTANCE OF		(CO-OPERATION]	__
RESPONSIBILITIES	__	SUBORDINATE RELATIONS	__
ADAPTABILITY TO CHANGES	__	SUPERVISOR RELATIONS	__
SUPERVISORY CAPABILITIES	__	**SAFETY**	__
LEADERSHIP AND DECISION		PERSONAL KNOWLEDGE	__
MAKING	__	APPLICATION	__
DELEGATION OF AUTHORITY	__	ATTITUDE	__
PLANNING, ORGANISING &			
CO-ORDINATING	__		

SUPERVISOR'S COMMENTS

STRONG POINTS	AREAS FOR IMPROVEMENT

POTENTIAL

EMPLOYEE'S COMMENTS

Figure 4.1 *Sample System 1 Performance appraisal record*

SECTION 1: PRESENT DUTIES

Assess the appraisee's performance in the areas listed using the following key:

A = Excellent – standards well above normally expected performance
B = Very good – standards better than normally expected performance
C = Good – meets normally expected performance
D = Satisfactory performance – development needed to overcome minor weaknesses
E = Poor – performance shows some significant weaknesses
F = Very poor – performance well below acceptable level

1. TECHNICAL/PROFESSIONAL KNOWLEDGE: A B C D E F
   Comments   ☐ ☐ ☐ ☐ ☐ ☐

2. APPROACH TO WORK: A B C D E F
   Comments   ☐ ☐ ☐ ☐ ☐ ☐

3. STAFF MANAGEMENT: A B C D E F
   Comments   ☐ ☐ ☐ ☐ ☐ ☐

4. INTERPERSONAL SKILLS: A B C D E F
   Comments   ☐ ☐ ☐ ☐ ☐ ☐

5. COMMUNICATION SKILLS: A B C D E F
   Comments   ☐ ☐ ☐ ☐ ☐ ☐

6. NUMERICAL/COMPUTER SKILLS: A B C D E F
   Comments   ☐ ☐ ☐ ☐ ☐ ☐

OVERALL ASSESSMENT

Give your assessment of the appraisee's overall performance.

Performance well above that normally expected	☐	Fully acceptable	☐
Not quite good enough on present performance	☐	Definitely unsatisfactory on present performance	☐

SECTION 2: POTENTIAL/CAREER PROGRESSION

Assess the appraisee's promotion potential by ticking the appropriate box.

Ready for higher-level work now   ☐

Has potential for higher-level work but needs further development   ☐

Unlikely to become capable of higher level work   ☐

Comments

Figure 4.2   *Sample System 2 Appraisal record (extract)*

First, although the marks A–F are explained in a key, the mere use of these letters is reminiscent of school reports and the scales they use. All too easily D is seen as a poor mark, whereas in fact it is a recognition that there is some scope for development. It is quite possible, and probably normal, to perform generally satisfactorily or even well in an area, while nonetheless still being able to benefit from further development. This particular problem is exacerbated because, after examining each of the performance areas, the appraiser is expected to make an overall assessment. If someone's performance is overall 'fully acceptable', appraisers may be unwilling to use the D scale to identify development needs. This is in spite of the fact that there is intended to be no mathematically weighted link between marks in each performance area and those given in the overall assessment. Quite sensibly this system avoids using the same scale for 'performance areas' as for 'overall performance'. Nonetheless many appraisers still make the connection. In other similar systems where the same scale is used both for 'performance areas' and 'overall performance' the danger of compounding this error must be greater.

A related problem occurs when one of the performance areas is not relevant to the job being appraised. The supporting documentation states quite sensibly that no mark can be given for this performance area. Unfortunately many appraisers get hung up on the need for mathematical weighting and feel the need to give a neutral C score!

In defence of this particular system, the overall assessment follows an analysis by performance areas rather than vice versa. This limits the danger of the 'halo' and 'horns' effects. The 'halo' effect occurs when the appraiser has an overall favourable impression of the appraisee and marks all areas of performance to fit this impression. The 'horns' effect is when the overall impression is unfavourable and the process is reversed.

There are other problems with the scale used in this system. Although the explanatory key spells out the marks as 'fully meets expected performance' etc, there is confusion as to what is meant by 'expected performance'. The designer's intention was that performance should be assessed against what would be expected of an *experienced job holder* in the position.

Unfortunately many appraisers misinterpret this and assess performance against their expectation of the *individual concerned*. This means that the learning curve is discounted and that someone new to a job may be marked as 'well above normally expected performance'. The result is an inadequate analysis of development needs. An additional pitfall is that managers assess their staff against each other. In one particular case, a personnel officer whose computer skills exceeded the requirements of the job was marked down because her manager didn't feel he couldn't give her a higher mark than colleagues who were computer specialists. The appraiser had failed to recognise that the specialists' skills needed to be assessed against the requirements of *their* jobs and that the personnel officer's skills needed to be assessed against the requirements of her job.

Sample System 2 also includes a section assessing potential. This is a useful point at which to make a few comments about the processes involved.

1. Potential needs to be assessed against the requirements of the higher level job and not performance of current duties. Although current performance will give some clue, don't make the mistake of thinking that someone who is excellent in their current job will necessarily be good at the duties of a higher level job.
2. Appraisees need to appreciate that recognising potential is not the same thing as offering promotion. Promotion can only be offered when a suitable opening is available.
3. Appraisees not reckoned suitable for higher level work are owed a detailed analysis of why and what they need to do to make themselves suitable for promotion (assuming that they are interested in career progression). Distinguish between two sets of needs – development to perform in the present job and development to provide for career progression.

Sample System 3

Sample System 3 is an 'output' system. It is concerned with specifying accountabilities, measuring how far these accountabilities have been met, and setting new goals for the next period. In our example (see Figure 4.3) we've shown the documentation completed for a publications officer whose job

---

PERFORMANCE APPRAISAL FORM

JOB HOLDER: Aisha Mohammed **APPRAISAL PERIOD:** April 1992 to March 1993

JOB TITLE Publications Officer

JOB PURPOSE: To manage the production, sale and distribution of the Trust's Publications

---

ACCOUNTABILITY 1   45 % of job   Rating _____

Sub-edit, design and ensure suitable production of the Trust's publications and training aids, within allocated resources.

Indicators

Quality, timeliness and cost effectiveness of Publications and training aids, as rated by manager.

Goals for next year

Provide proposals for publications project for the year. Produce six new major print publications in 1993/94

Assumptions/constraints

Availability of money for speculative investment output from Research Department.

Figure 4.3   *Sample System 3 Performance appraisal form (extract)*

ACCOUNTABILITY 2 15 % of job Rating ___

Distribute stocks of publications and training aids to the Trust's offices, Control central stocks, re-order stocks as required.

Indicators

Efficient stock distribution and control, as rated by manager.

Goals for next year

Ensure that new system of central despatch operate efficiently.

Assumptions/constraints

ACCOUNTABILITY 3 10 % of job Rating ___

Co-ordinate sales and stock reporting process, highlight points for attention by Manager.

Indicators

Quality and timeliness of management information provided, as rated by Manager.

Goals for next year

Produce quarterly investment recovery reports.

Assumptions/constraints

Figure 4.3 *Continued*

ACCOUNTABILITY 4   <u>20</u> % of job   Rating ____

Publicise availability of Trust's saleable titles, stimulate sales by direct mail, advertising, review design and produce promotional material, within allocated resources.

Measures

Suitability of material designed as rated by Manager.

Goals for next year

Execute specific promotions.

Assumptions/constraints

Production of materials for promotion

ACCOUNTABILITY 5   <u>10</u> % of job   Rating ____

Draft for approval of Director press releases, as required, produce and distribute press releases.

Measures

The quality of press releases as rated by Director, their timeliness.

Goals for next year

Assumptions/constraints

Figure 4.3 *Continued*

involves managing a small publications department. Her responsibilities involve producing, selling and distributing her organisation's books and training aids. It could be argued that some of the performance measures specified by her appraiser are rather woolly and very subjective. The same also applies to the goals set which are not accompanied by the kind of measures which would be useful later in assessing the extent to which those goals have been achieved. In Chapter 7 we will discuss how to set valid objectives and output measures.

Meanwhile, one of the features of this system worth noting is that it gives a weighting to each of the principal accountabilities in the job. This is useful particularly where an overall assessment of performance is to be made. Clearly some areas of a job are not as important as others. In appraising staff, you've got to be careful not to allow failure or shortcomings in one relatively minor area to weigh disproportionately in your view of that person's performance as a whole. Even if your system doesn't explicitly ask you to put percentages against each element of the job, this is still a mental process worth following. Also useful is that the assumptions and constraints relating to the achievement of 'goals' are made explicit.

Sample System 4

System 3's main failing is that it doesn't provide a framework for the analysis of 'inputs'. This problem is addressed by Sample System 4 (see Figure 4.4) which combines elements of both the input and output approaches. It starts with a review of previous objectives and the extent to which they've been achieved: it proceeds with an analysis of strengths and weaknesses, and it concludes by setting objectives for the next period.

System 4 goes some way towards offsetting the problems encountered with System 2. Instead of an A–F marking we have a scale which is explicitly established to identify development needs. It's also made clear that not all the performance areas listed are necessarily relevant, and that other unspecified areas can and should be added to the analysis. Unfortunately the form design leaves only a very limited amount of space for comments to explain the reasons for marks and why development is required. Again, this can reduce the appraisal to a box ticking exercise as we saw in

SECTION 1. REVIEW OF PREVIOUS YEAR'S OBJECTIVES
Complete and append Section 3 of last year's appraisal record.

SECTION 2. ANALYSIS OF STRENGTHS AND AREAS FOR DEVELOPMENT

St = Strength – exceeds requirements

Sf = Satisfactory – meets expectations

Dv = Development needed

N = Not part of present job

PERFORMANCE AREA	St	Sf	Dv	N	COMMENT
1. Job Knowledge					
2. Accuracy/Quality					
3. Planning					
4. Organisation					
5. Cost Control					
6. Communication					
7. Decision Making					
8. Delegation					
9. Supervision					
10. Interpersonal skills					
11.					
12.					
13.					

Figure 4.4 *Sample System 4 Sample appraisal record (extract)*

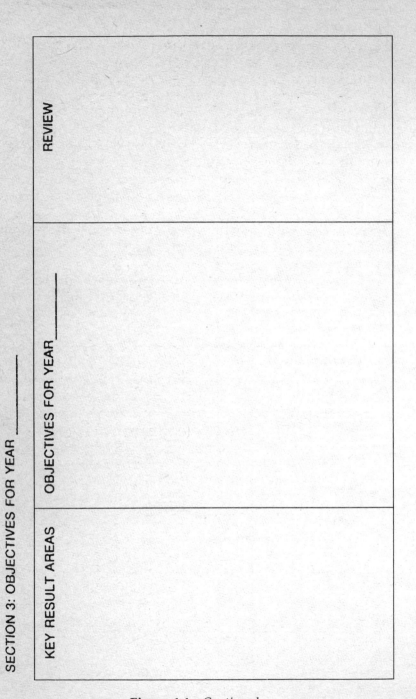

Figure 4.4 *Continued*

System 1. Appraisal is intended to be a process of analysis. You must ask yourself 'What exactly do I mean by strength in oral communication" or satisfactory decision making"?' This point is taken up again in Chapter 8 where the 'key questions' approach to performance analysis is described.

One last point to make about System 4's analysis of 'inputs' is that it associates performance very closely with the strengths and development needs of the individual. It fails to make clear that an important part of performance analysis should be an examination of blockages to effective performance. As we've said, these go beyond the individual's weaknesses and involve issues such as resourcing, relationships with the boss and so forth. This point is further developed in the next chapter.

System 4's emphasis on 'outputs' brings us to the issues of setting and measuring of objectives, which will be dealt with in Chapter 7. At this point, however, it is worth noting that the 'objectives' in System 4 are derived from 'key results areas'. If you operate such a system yourself, then a first step must be to clarify what is meant by 'key result areas'. These should be described in the job description, but in practice many job descriptions are rather inadequate. Often they are drawn up for purposes of recruitment and then almost forgotten. Good appraisal systems often require appraiser and appraisee to review and update the job description as a preliminary to appraisal. As appraiser you may find that you have to go even further and review the structure of the job description so that the job purpose, main responsibilities and attendant key result areas are clearly identified.

Sample System 5

Sample System 5 is an example of a narrative report. It demonstrates the flexibility which such systems can have. However, while there is the danger that scale systems may reduce appraisal to a box ticking exercise, narrative systems depend upon the appraisers' ability and willingness to express themselves in writing. Narrative formats can also make it difficult to compare appraisees with each other. Such comparisons may be necessary if decisions are to be made as to who is, and who isn't, eligible for a performance-related

1. Main priorities agreed for the period up to the next appraisal interview.

2. Significant changes desired, either to the job, the structure or working methods, which will help the post holder improve on current performance.

Figure 4.5 *Sample System 5 Appraisal record (extract)*

3. Training and development recommendations related to the post holder's present or possible future role.

4. Any further points which have emerged from the interview which require further action.

Figure 4.5 *Continued*

pay (PRP) reward. One appraiser may use the phrase 'very good' where another might say 'excellent' or 'remarkable' to mean the same thing. Narrative approaches do, however, allow a fuller explanation of an appraiser's reasonings and a greater opportunity to incorporate the views of the appraisee.

Appraisee preparation and documentation

None of the examples reviewed above has included any documentation for the appraisee to complete, either by way of preparation for the appraisal discussion or by way of contributing to the record of that discussion. As the success of appraisal depends upon maximising the involvement of the appraisee and giving him/her a sense of ownership, this omission can be a serious shortcoming in system design. Fortunately, in recent years, many organisations implementing or reforming appraisal have taken account of this factor and incorporated appropriate features in their design.

One example of this is the growing use of pre-appraisal forms. As part of appraisal documentation, appraisees are provided with a form to complete prior to the discussion. In some schemes this is purely for the appraisees' personal and private use, helping them to consolidate their thoughts and prepare for the discussion. In other schemes, the completed pre-appraisal form is intended to be submitted to the appraiser in advance so that he/she can have some prior indication of the issues of concern to the appraisee. This can cause a problem if the appraisee is reluctant to pre-warn the appraiser or if the appraiser looks at the appraisee's views without first examining their own perceptions independently. In other words, there is a danger that the appraiser's views can be prejudiced by the appraisee's views.

Some designs require both appraisee and appraiser to complete pre-appraisal forms but leave it to the discretion of both parties as to whether they swap forms in advance. If this is a feature of your system, you need to decide how you're going to operate it. If it is not currently part of your formal system, you may decide in consultation with your staff that it might be beneficial to use something like it within your own department. Whatever you do, preparation both by appraisers and appraisees is one of the keys to good appraisal.

If completed documentation is to be a matter of record and is to be seen by a third party, it's also reasonable to allow the appraisee the opportunity to record their own comments. Some systems simply require the appraisee to sign the completed forms, but appraisees may feel a sense of coercion and that their signature might be taken as agreement with their manager's assessment. The opportunity to record their own views, perhaps pointing out anything which their appraiser has overlooked or possibly distorted, is usually valued by appraisees. Even if your system doesn't prescribe this, you might still consider offering the appraisee the opportunity to write comments which you can append to the formal documentation.

1. Personnel issues documentation to appraiser/manager

2. Appraiser agrees time for meeting with appraisee, giving at least 7 days notice and issues pre-appraisal form

3A. Appraisee completes pre-appraisal form and gathers thoughts	3B. Appraiser completes pre-appraisal form and gathers thoughts

4. Appraiser and appraisee meet for structured appraisal discussion

5. Appraiser completes documentation and submits to appraisee for written comments and signature

6. Appraiser and appraisee retain copies of completed documentation. Appraiser submits one copy to the 'two-up' manager

7. 'Two-up' manager reviews, adds comments, if necessary takes action on an exception basis, and returns the form to personnel

Figure 4.6 *Sample appraisal process*

5 *Improving appraisee performance*

Improving appraisee performance is one of the prime objectives of appraisal. Therefore, as an appraiser, you need to examine those factors which determine, or limit, performance and think about what you can do to help your staff perform more effectively.

In broad terms, performance will be limited by:

- the skills and knowledge of the appraisee;
- the resources available;
- the quality and style of management provided;
- the appraisee's level of motivation and the extent to which the job suits them.

Skills and knowledge

It's an obvious point that an individual's performance will be constrained by any lack of skill or knowledge required by the job. Indeed, much of the appraisal process may be geared to diagnosing skills and knowledge areas which require development. Distinguish between a lack of ability and a lack of aptitude. If someone lacks ability but has the aptitude, then what is needed is training. If, on the other hand, someone lacks aptitude, training will not help that person develop the requisite skills. In such a case, action should involve re-examining job design to see how the abilities and aptitudes of the appraisee has can be best utilised – round holes for round pegs.

Furthermore, it's important to avoid falling into the trap of thinking that all performance problems have a training solution. It's all too easy to boil the appraisal process down to 'what courses do you fancy?'. There is a danger that thinking about training provision precedes rather than follows from an analysis of training needs – the cart being put before the horse.

Sometimes managers use training as a way of avoiding responsibility – it becomes a 'cop out', allowing blame to be passed onto the shortcomings of the appraisee. By the same token, the appraisee may feel that the real issue has been missed.

Jack complains 'I've got too much work to do. I can't meet the deadlines.' Jill, his boss, replies, 'You've got to learn to manage your time. I'll send you on a time-management course.' Jack doesn't see it that way. For him the problem lies in resources: 'The organisation is simply expecting too much from one person.' He also believes that some of the difficulty is created by Jill and her failure to prioritise and communicate. If Jack goes on a time-management course in this frame of mind, it's unlikely to be very useful. This is not simply because the training might not be addressing the real problem; it's because Jack wants to prove that it can't. 'There's nothing wrong with me. I haven't got anything to learn and there's nothing I can do about it anyway. Jill's the one who needs to go on a course.'

We also need to recognise that training is subject to the law of diminishing returns. This law states that in any productive process if one input is increased while others are kept constant, there comes a point where returns on that input diminish. Just as you can't increase agricultural yield by putting more and more fertiliser on the same piece of land, so there comes a point where the return on training will diminish if other resources are not increased proportionately.

Resources

The last point reminds us that performance will be limited if the resources available are inadequate for the task. These resources may be in the form of equipment, office space, support staff, budgetary control, access to technology and/or information. Although organisations spend a lot of money on employing people, sometimes they fail to provide those people with adequate resources to make them fully productive. As an appraiser you need to explore the extent to which a lack of resources inhibits your appraisee's performance. Your ability to supply increased resources may be limited by your position in the organisation or other economic constraints. However, one of the key roles of a team manager is to act as the team's ambassador to more senior management and to fight for the resources the team needs and can justify.

The quality of management

This may be one of the hardest issues for some appraisers to deal with. After all, it requires them to investigate the extent to which they themselves may be responsible for inhibiting an appraisee's performance.

These inhibiting factors can take a number of forms. They might include an inappropriate management style which could be too *laissez-faire* for someone who needs clearer direction, or too structured for someone who needs greater leeway. The problem could be a failure to make and communicate decisions. It could be a tendency to interrupt constantly or to interfere, or to re-jig priorities. Sometimes it's a matter of too willingly taking on work from above and dumping it too easily on those below. The problem may be a failure to show adequate interest in the appraisee's work or to appreciate some of the difficulties involved.

As we said in Chapter 2, one of the main benefits of appraisal is that it provides the appraiser with an opportunity to receive feedback on his/her management style. Unless you establish an open and frank relationship this feedback may not be forthcoming. Engage the appraisee's help to identify changes you might need to make to your way of managing.

Unfortunately not all appraisal systems place this aspect of performance development explicitly on the agenda. This is one of those situations in which you may find that to make appraisal work for you and your staff you have to go beyond the minimalist requirements of the system.

The appraisee's motivation

One of the main determinants of performance is the appraisee's motivation. If you are to enhance the performance of your staff, then you need to understand, and pay due regard to, the factors which can affect motivation. In particular, you need to uncover anything which may create a sense of dissatisfaction within their job.

Here is not the place for a full review of motivation theory. However, I have always found Herzberg's 'Hygiene Factor' and 'Expectancy' theories particularly useful in the appraisal context. These are examined below. In Chapter 6 I extend this discussion to look at how values, needs and personality impact on motivation.

Herzberg's Hygiene Factor Theory

Herzberg identified two distinct sets of factors affecting motivation. One set he called 'motivators': these are the factors which relate to job satisfaction. The other set he called 'hygiene factors': these are the factors which potentially produce dissatisfaction.

In Herzberg's model the motivators are:

- achievement
- recognition
- the work itself
- responsibility
- advancement/growth.

The hygiene factors are:

- company policy and administration
- supervision
- working conditions
- interpersonal relations
- salary
- status
- job security.

According to Herzberg, the importance of a 'hygiene' factor is felt only when it is absent. An employee will take good working conditions for granted, but these will not give him/her any particular job satisfaction. On the other hand, bad working conditions are usually a source of dissatisfaction. Therefore, adverse hygiene factors demotivate, but when they are good they have only a neutral effect and are not sufficient to produce positive motivation. This point is illustrated by the expressions on the three faces in Figure 5.1.

The implications for you as an appraising manager are twofold.

1. *You need to look for adverse hygiene factors and see what can be done to tackle them.*
   - 'Are poor physical working conditions a source of dissatisfaction?'
   - 'Is there a problem in the interpersonal relations between the appraisee and his colleagues?'
   - 'Are there problems in the way I relate to her as a supervisor?'

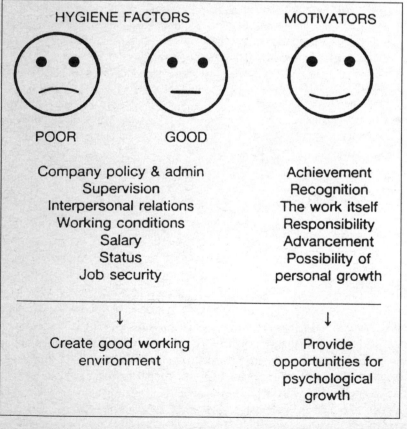

Figure 5.1   *Herzberg's hygiene factors and motivators*

- 'Is company policy, or the administration system with its bureaucratic impositions, a demotivating force and can I do anything to improve it or limit the damage?'

2. *You need to examine the motivators and issues of job design.*
Does the job as presently constituted provide scope for the individual to obtain achievement, recognition, responsibility and growth? One of the objectives of the appraisal should be to explore what staff feel about their jobs, the scope they offer and the ways in which they might be 'enriched' to provide for greater job satisfaction.

Herzberg places a lot of emphasis on the concept of 'job enrichment'. Job enrichment does not mean piling one undemanding task on top of another or switching from one undemanding task to another. It means looking for 'vertical job development' rather than 'horizontal job expansion'.

These terms 'vertical job development' and 'horizontal job expansion' require some explanation and illustration. A horizontally designed job involves an individual executing a narrow range of tasks on an often repeated basis, contributing one small part towards the completion of the product or the provision of the service as a whole. A vertically designed job involves the individual in doing a wide range of tasks and contributing a greater share to the complete product or service.

This oft-quoted example comes from a motor manufacturing plant. Originally jobs were horizontally designed: every time a chassis came past on the assembly line a fitter fitted a particular bolt and so on, fitting bolts on to partly made cars all day. Then the jobs were redesigned in a vertical fashion. Instead of doing a single repetitive task to a large number of cars, fitters now worked in small teams building cars together, each one doing a wider range of tasks and seeing the completed (or more nearly completed) car develop in front of their eyes. The result was not only a more varied and interesting job, but also a greater sense of responsibility for, and pride in, the completed product.

This kind of job redesign has, of course, major implications for capital investment and it is unlikely that as a line manager you would be in a position to implement change of such proportions! Note also that, although this kind of change may lead to greater job satisfaction for employees, it doesn't necessarily mean greater productivity as it may involve under-utilising specialists' skills and equipment. Indeed, the motor manufacturer referred to above later shifted back to a more traditional assembly line approach.

However, the point being made here is that many jobs do lend themselves to some form of redesign. Take, for instance, the clerical functions carried out by a commercial training organisation. These include:

- responding to customer enquiries;
- taking bookings;
- invoicing customers;
- liaising with course venues and arranging equipment;
- duplicating handout materials;
- liaising with the course presenter;

and so forth. If the scale of operation allows, there are two ways of approaching these tasks. Either one person can be responsible for a single clerical function across all of the courses, or one person can be responsible for all of the clerical functions in respect of a single course (or group of courses). The former would be horizontal design, the latter is vertical. Again, the vertical design gives greater variety, greater responsibility (and therefore concern for quality) and greater scope for a sense of achievement.

As an appraiser you need to look for such opportunities for job redesign and discuss these with your appraisees. Your aim should be to create jobs which are more fulfilling and motivating.

Expectancy Theory

Herzberg's theory presents only one of the ways of looking at motivation and provides only part of the picture. Another part of that picture is provided by what is known as 'Expectancy Theory'. Historically, motivation theories have concentrated on 'needs'. If someone has a need they are motivated to fulfil it. However, 'need' is not always sufficient to motivate someone to do something – they have to believe that the effort will lead to the need being fulfilled. Let's look at an example.

Bill is a sales executive with a photocopier company. His boss tells him that if he succeeds in getting sales up to £X,000, he will be in line for the new job of sales manager to be created later that year. The job offers a higher salary, better car and increased responsibility. Will Bill work harder?

The answer is he will work harder, but only if the following apply:

- _He feels that by working harder he will increase sales and meet the target._ There is no motivation for Bill to increase his call rate unless he believes that an increased call rate will lead to adequately increased sales.
- _He believes that if he does achieve the sales target, he will get promotion._ Bill may not believe what his boss says; or think that the creation of the new post is unlikely; or recognise that, when it comes to it, the job is likely go to someone with more management experience.
- _He values promotion sufficiently._ Bill may like his current lifestyle and not want the responsibility or changes involved in a new job. He may want promotion and be attracted to the idea of the higher salary, better car and increased responsibility, but he may feel that these rewards are not sufficiently valuable to put in the amount of extra effort needed to achieve them.

The implication is that you shouldn't assume that any reward you offer an appraisee will necessarily motivate him/her to work harder or learn new skills. Don't make vague promises which aren't, or can't, be fulfilled. This can lead to a situation in which an appraisee has little faith in the carrots you offer. Not only do you have to examine whether an increase in effort could actually achieve the target set, and whether the appraisee is likely to see the reward as worth the effort, you also have to recognise that your credibility is essential. Recognise also that not everyone would make the same calculations as you would.

6 Performance, personality and preferences

In the last chapter we looked at some of the factors affecting appraisee motivation and the practical implications of these for you as an appraising manager. The approach was essentially a general one, although we did recognise differences between individuals in the way they may calculate the relationship between the rewards and efforts. In this chapter I want to explore further the differences which exist between individual appraisees.

Personality differences and behaviour

In managing and in appraising your staff you're involved in dealing with a number of different characters. The differences between individuals are what make them unique or special, and an individual's special characteristics, taken together, constitute what we call their 'personality'. Personality manifests itself in, and influences, behaviour. Personality therefore impacts upon the way individual appraisees perform at work and the preferences they have for certain tasks and jobs. Therefore as an appraiser you need to be attuned to the implications of differences in personality if you are to help your staff perform effectively. This is particularly important if you are to provide them with the tasks and jobs which make the most of their talents and tap their individual motivations. In other words, as an appraiser wanting to get the best out of people, it's important for you to understand what makes each member of your staff tick.

In understanding the complexity of individuals and 'what makes them tick', we often resort to stereotyping to make sense of what would otherwise be a baffling diversity. But even if the use of stereotyping is inevitable, we must be careful to avoid its crudest excesses. Individuals cannot be divided into five or six simple personality types from which their behaviour can be easily or consistently determined. Always bear in mind the limitations of any stereotypes and realise that they are only generalisations, otherwise people may surprise you by acting in a way that falls outside the scope of your predictions.

Psychologists differ in their views on what constitutes the basis of personality. Some see it as a product of innate or biological factors. Some emphasise the determining effects of early life experiences. Others regard personality as a complex interaction between genetic, social and environmental factors. Psychologists also differ in their views as to how fixed personality is. By definition they'll agree that personality relates to 'enduring traits', but they'll disagree as to what they mean by 'enduring'. At issue here is the scope that each of us has to choose our own actions and the extent to which they are predetermined by our fixed personalities. This is an important subject in both psychology and philosophy, but not one appropriate for debate here. Suffice it to say that even if an individual cannot change the fundamentals of their personality, they might still be able to alter or modify certain of their behaviour patterns. This ability can be important in adjusting to different work situations. For instance, someone who was once very cautious about decision making can change into someone more prepared to take risks and make decisions if that is what is required by their job.

Of course, certain patterns of behaviour go deep and may only be changed with difficulty. These tend to be the patterns of behaviour which have been learnt early in life and reinforced by experience. If behaving in a certain way brought a reward (maybe the recognition of a parent, teacher, a boss or friend) then the individual is more likely to apply that pattern of behaviour again. If behaving in another way led to some form of punishment (disapproval, deprivation, frustration) then the individual is likely to avoid that pattern of behaviour in future.

It's easy to get into behaviour patterns which dig out a 'rut'.

That is, the more often someone behaves in a certain way, the more likely it is that they will go on behaving in that way and the less easy it is for them to get out of the 'rut' and behave in a different way.

As an appraiser you need to be attuned to the patterns of behaviour with which individual appraisees feel comfortable and to be aware of the satisfactions they derive and the anxieties they suffer. These satisfactions and anxieties relate in turn to the needs and values of the individuals concerned – and account for the way they behave and perform at work. Let's look also at some of the practical implications these may have for you in managing individual appraisees.

Stability/change

One important set of differences between individuals is the extent to which one individual values stability or, alternatively, relishes change.

We live in a climate of rapid change. Some individuals find adjustment to change difficult and painful. Change can mean uncertainty, unpredictability and a loss of control – such people have a high need for stability. For others change means challenge, growth, opportunity and variety.

If change is required then you need to handle individuals with high stability needs carefully. Show them why change is necessary, allay their fears as to the implications of change, and help them to see that their contribution continues to be valued.

With those who have a high need for change, you may need to restrain their enthusiasm and emphasise to them the value of stable processes and piecemeal reform. As far as possible, provide these people with variety in their jobs enabling them to move on from one project to another. Be careful, though, that their desire to move on doesn't lead them to leave jobs unfinished. With these individuals you may either have to emphasise the need to complete jobs, or structure the jobs so that they can hand over the final stages to someone more adept at completing. Be aware that there are many people around who are very good at taking a job to 85 per cent completion, but who find it very difficult to finish off as their high need for change and variety takes over.

Structure/leeway

By the need for structure, I mean the need to operate within clear guidelines and instructions. The need for leeway means the need of the individual to be free to determine how he/she approaches a job. Some people like to be given precise instructions; others find instructions irksome.

People with high structure needs perform well on tasks which can be routinised and where adherence to procedure is important. Often they are good at paying meticulous attention to detail. It is difficult for someone with high leeway needs to feel motivated by these sorts of tasks. Their strength lies instead in dealing with tasks which cannot be so easily routinised and where discretion is important. They have a higher tolerance of ambiguity. They have a greater willingness to accept approximations and imperfections than does the individual with the high structure needs who will tend to value precision and perfection.

There is always a danger that an individual who places low emphasis on precision will become slapdash. On the other hand there is the danger that the individual who places a high value on perfection will get bogged down in detail and invest disproportionate efforts to achieve marginal improvements. As an appraiser you need both to value the contribution which each type of person makes, and also help individuals to recognise when they should pay more attention to detail and when they need to be prepared to deal in wider generalities.

Certainty/risk

These two dimensions are closely related to the structure/leeway dimensions. A need for certainty will involve a cautious approach to decision making, or indeed an avoidance of decision making. Such people need to be encouraged to take more risks and certainly shouldn't be punished for sub-optimal decisions. A high need for, or a tolerance of, risk may lead to snap decisions in which options are not properly examined. While in some circumstances it may be appropriate to make decisions quickly, decision makers always need to assess the situation and the kind of decision making required.

Again, as an appraiser you need to help your staff recognise their own propensities and to help them develop their understanding of the decision-making process.

High/low social needs

While everyone may have some social needs, there is clearly quite a difference in the extent to which individuals feel these needs. Some people are obviously more socially orientated than others. This may affect not only their interpersonal skills, but also their preference for different working patterns.

Social needs can be looked at under three headings. These are:

- the need to belong to a group;
- the need for a variety of social contact;
- the need to be liked.

Belonging to a group

For many people the need to belong to a desirable group is a strong motivator. They will do what is needed to gain the acceptance of that group and perform to avoid exclusion or expulsion. In these circumstances team pressures often work well to produce performance – individual team members don't want to let the side down or lose face in front of peers. However, for these pressures to be effective, the team has to be one to which the individual wishes to belong – team membership has to be desirable.

To be a good manager and team leader, you need to work on building team spirit and creating an affinity between team members. This may involve a range of team-building tactics which lie beyond the scope of this book but which include activities such as outward bound training, charity walks, socials or simply lunching together. Identify the needs which individuals have to be part of a team and try to provide them with the opportunities to which they will respond. Young people often have a particularly strong need for belonging to a group. Where possible, it's important to integrate them within a team rather than leaving them to work in isolation.

However, you must also be aware that some individuals don't feel such a strong need to belong and some may even be irked by too much 'team building'. If you have to manage 'non-team' people in a situation where team working is important, encourage these people to take part, but remember you may put them off by making unreasonable demands for out of hours socialising or weekend activities.

Variety of social contact

Some people, whether or not they have strong needs to belong to a group, like to have a lot of social contact, mixing with a variety of people, enjoying brief relationships with them. Such people, often classified as extrovert, make good sales and customer-facing staff. These people can also get very bored if they are stuck in the office or factory not meeting new people. Try to provide these types with the opportunity to get out of the office or factory at least from time to time. Going to conferences, exhibitions or on field trips can be very stimulating for them.

Others, and these may often be people with high stability needs, do not like meeting new people and prefer instead secure, certain and established relationships. If you are considering changing the structure of a job or someone's role remember that such people may feel threatened if any changes you propose to their new responsibilities involve them in dealings with new people.

The need to be liked

Most people like to be liked and appreciated. This need is, however, stronger for some than for others. Some people are thicker skinned than others and will pursue their ends whatever impact this may have on people's opinion of them. Others have a high need for affection, particularly from the boss. Such people may look to you as a kind of 'big brother/sister' or 'parent figure' and need your constant and explicit approval. It's important to give these people your time, attention and consideration – a special personal relationship. The appraisal itself is an opportunity for you to meet this need by giving your time and attention to individual members of staff.

Short-/long-term 'achievement needs'

Many people identify 'achievement' as their main source of job satisfaction and motivation. There are, of course, differences as to how people mark their achievement. For some, achievement is marked by monetary reward or status symbols. For others, value is placed upon explicit recognition from the boss or customer. For yet others, achievement satisfaction comes from self-awareness that a job's been done well. These differences will account for the ways in which individuals respond to rewards and may affect your strategy for motivating them.

While most people have this need to achieve, it's important to recognise that some will be looking for short-term achievement and will need quick results, while others may be happier to wait for the gratification of their achievement needs. This means that some people can be highly motivated by the challenge of tackling a large complex assignment. Others may find the length of timescale a problem, gaining their 'buzz' instead from attacking and completing a number of short-term tasks which have rapid pay-offs.

One of the motivational problems of working on long-term projects is that although considerable effort may be required, ultimate achievement is uncertain – nine months down the road the project might be shelved. People working on long-term projects may still need short-term achievement satisfaction. Design projects to build in achievement 'milestones' which can be celebrated as the project progresses. Thus, long before completion, the project is associated with a sense of achievement and success which carries it through.

Of course, there are many more dimensions to people's value systems and the ways in which they behave. This brief discussion will have made you sensitive to that diversity and the need to adopt a strategy particular to the needs of each individual. I hope this discussion will also have alerted you to the danger of assuming that everyone is motivated by the same things that motivate you. This is a mistake which many managers make, expecting others to be motivated as they are (perhaps by career progression, or the intellectual fascination of the job) and being frustrated and uncomprehending when staff do not seem to be motivated by such stimuli.

7 Setting and agreeing objectives

I mentioned in Chapter 3, 'Which Appraisal System?', that many systems involve both setting objectives and monitoring, or measuring, performance against them. If you're an appraiser facing this requirement, you may already be aware of how much more difficult this is to do in practice than it may appear in principle. It could be argued that setting objectives is such a difficult task and standards of objective setting vary so widely from manager to manager that it's best not to have an appraisal system which places too much emphasis upon objectives. That, however, is an argument for personnel specialists and systems designers. As an appraiser you may have no choice but to work with an objective setting system. I hope, therefore, that this chapter will clarify the issues for you and help you to use objective setting in a meaningful way.

It seems to me that there are three broad areas of difficulty. These are:

- understanding what is meant by an objective;
- expressing objectives in relevant, specific and meaningful ways;
- relating the achievement (or non-achievement) of specified objectives to overall performance.

What is meant by an 'objective'?

You may have encountered what, to my mind, is a rather tedious debate to distinguish 'aims' from 'objectives'. In this debate, 'aims' are seen as fairly broad while 'objectives' are seen as specific. Although personnel specialists might find it useful to make such a distinction, attaching technical meaning to everyday words often 'muddies the water' and creates confusion. If you look up 'aim' and 'objective' in the *Concise Oxford English Dictionary*, you'll see that they are defined in terms of each other. Distinguishing between them, as far as everyday English is concerned, is thus a semantic nonsense. Even if we do accept that a technical meaning can be attached to these words, a problem still remains – how specific does an 'aim' have to be to qualify as an 'objective'? This can't be a simple black and white distinction – there are degrees of 'specificity' and some objectives will be more specific than others. I suggest below that the real issue is not whether a particular statement qualifies as an 'objective' or is merely an 'aim', but whether it can be made more usable by tightening it against a set of criteria for 'good objectives'.

Another confusion is between different kinds of objective. I distinguish three types:

1 *Projects or progress tasks which are one-off initiatives to meet the team or corporate plan.* For example, 'set up a distance learning centre' or 'produce a new catalogue'.
2. *Standards of service or activity levels to be met on a continuing basis.* An example of this might be 'answer the telephone promptly' or 'make ten field visits per week'.
3. *Actions to improve performance.* Examples might include 'attend a course on spreadsheets', 'check stock levels with Jack before placing new orders' or even (and I have seen this on an appraisal form) 'arrive on time for work'.

There's no reason why each of these three types should not be considered as valid. I would suggest, however, that there is a tendency for appraisers and appraisees to focus on only one type of objective. As a result they fail to explore the contribution which could be made by the other types. In principle, there's no reason an individual's set of objectives could not include all three types. There will be differences between different sorts of job. A managerial or executive role may allow more scope for project type objectives. A role which is characterised by routine or 'maintenance' tasks may need to make more use of 'service standards' or 'activity level' type objectives.

The point also has to be made that not all objectives are equal. The objective of 'arrive on time for work' may be a necessity but it is hardly a sufficient condition of good performance. It would be unfair to judge the person for whom 'arrive on time' had been set as an objective (and who had fully complied) against someone whose punctuality was not an issue and who had been set, but failed, to meet the objective of (say) answering all customer correspondence within two working days. We'll return to this point later when we consider how to relate achievement of objectives to overall performance.

Expressing objectives

The second difficulty I identified was in expressing objectives in relevant, specific and meaningful ways. Here the mnemonic 'SMART' may help. SMART stands for 'Specific, Measurable, Agreed, Realistic, and Timed' and is used to help appraisers think about the characteristics of a good objective. These criteria provide a basis for tightening objectives and making them more useful. Always ask yourself 'Can I make this objective "Smarter"?'

Let's look at each of the criteria in turn.

S = Specific

This means that an objective should be clearly expressed in a way which minimises the scope for differences in interpretation between appraiser and appraisee. Vague and wishy-washy statements won't do.

M = Measurable

Where possible and appropriate you should seek to establish quantifiable measures. Some tasks lend themselves to this process more easily than others. Sometimes objectives may be expressed as specific budget targets – sales revenue, costs, profit, return on investment and so forth. For instance, 'Expand sales of Superwidge to £X,000'; 'Reduce costs of stockholding by 10 per cent.' In doing this it's also important to express constraints. For instance, 'Reduce costs of stockholding by 10 per cent while maintaining established customer delivery terms.' Alternatively, objectives may be expressed in terms of a measurable level of service. An objective such as 'Reform system to optimise customer record services' could be refined as 'Reform system to ensure all priority A record requests are serviced within two hours and that all priority B record requests are serviced within eight hours.'

However, some outputs are less easy to quantify and it is often their qualitative dimensions which are critical. For instance, if the task is to produce a new brochure, then the meaningful measures are going to be qualitative rather than quantitative. There is an important point here. Because some managers want objective performance measures, they reject any objective that can't be expressed in quantifiable terms. The result can be that valuable objectives are ignored and unimportant objectives are incorporated simply because they lend themselves to favourable statistical analysis. Sometimes this means reducing objectives to activity level measures (ie the volume of work) without looking at the quality of work. The cliché, 'If you can't measure it, you can't manage it' shouldn't be taken as meaning 'only those tasks that are quantifiable are worth managing'.

A = Agreed

Objectives need to be agreed by both appraiser and appraisee. Although you need to give advance thought to what you think would make a sensible series of objectives, try to get suggestions coming from your appraisees so that they can take a lead in determining their own objectives. Remember also that 'compliance' is not the same as 'agreement'. Make sure that your staff are committed to achieving objectives they see as realistic, rather than merely going along with something they feel is imposed upon them by you.

R = Realistic

Every objective has to be achievable. Furthermore, the appraisee has to believe that it is achievable – otherwise he/she will feel swamped and demotivated. If someone is accountable for an objective, the achievement of the objective must lie within their power, or at the very least the appraisee's actions must be able to strongly influence whether or not it is achieved. If achieving an objective depends too heavily on factors outside the appraisee's control, then it becomes an unfair measure of performance.

Closely related to 'realistic' is the issue of resources. (It's tempting to introduce this as a second 'R' but to do so would upset the spelling of the mnemonic.) An objective can only be 'realistic' if it's 'resourced'. There's no point in agreeing objectives that cannot be achieved because the resources are not available.

The most important resource at an appraisee's disposal is probably his/her own time and the time of the team involved. Appraisees can be over-ambitious about the tasks and projects they think they can accomplish. They may lose sight of the fact that all their time can't be given to the execution of 'progress' tasks and that a greater proportion of their time needs to be reserved for 'maintenance' tasks. In agreeing objectives be careful to ensure that resources are adequate and have not already been committed elsewhere.

T = Timed

As well as deciding what needs to be done, timescales and completion dates need to be specified. A problem with an annual appraisal is that by default it may be assumed that objectives don't have to be achieved until the end of the appraisal period. This is clearly a nonsense.

In some circumstances, it may be difficult to set objectives for a whole year ahead. This is particularly true in a climate of instability or rapid change. A quarterly review may be necessary if the system is to work at all.

Two further criteria should be assessed. These are 'Integrated' and – the acid test – 'Worthwhile'.

I = Integrated

An individual's objectives need to be integrated with, and derived from, those of the organisation and department in which he/she works. They need also to be compatible with main responsibilities identified in the job description. If objectives are not integrated in this way, the individual may put effort into something which is not contributing towards departmental objectives and is outside the scope of the job. It's not good enough to allow the appraisee to choose objectives on an 'I fancy doing that' basis. Start with a statement of the departmental objectives and ask the appraisee to examine the contribution which he/she could make to these.

W = Worthwhile

This is a good final check. Even if an objective fits all the other criteria is it worth achieving? Is it worth, for instance, the effort and resources which will be required to achieve it? If the answer is 'no', it's not worthwhile and the objective should be rejected as inappropriate.

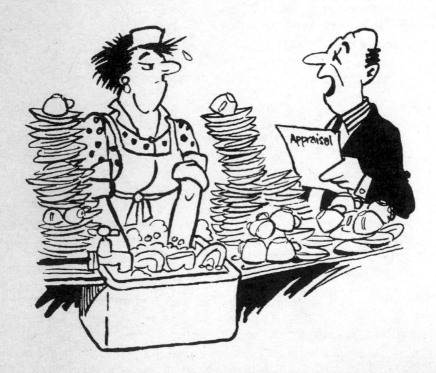

'Your objective for next year will be to wash 2,468,321 cups and saucers.'

The cartoon provides a humorous example of a poorly-set objective. It may be 'Specific' and 'Measurable', but it seems to be imposed rather than 'Agreed', it may not be 'Realistic' and it certainly isn't 'Time-based'. Its measurability is, in fact, part of its weakness and is likely to encourage cheating. Who's going to count the cups and saucers?

Relating achievement to overall performance

I've talked to many appraising managers who have found difficulty in relating achievement of objectives to some kind of overall performance assessment. I'm sure that the difficulty is often caused, or at least exacerbated, by poor guidance from their systems designers.

There are two related questions which the appraiser needs to address:

1. Does the achievement of objectives equate with good performance?
2. Does failure to achieve objectives equate with poor performance?

At first sight these questions may appear naive. Surely if someone has met their objectives, they've performed well. In fact, this is not necessarily so. Firstly the objectives may have been important, but not particularly demanding. Secondly, they may have been achieved despite, rather than because of, the efforts of the appraisee. If a sales executive, for example, makes or exceeds a sales target, this may be due to new initiatives by the marketing department, an upturn in the economy, or difficulties encountered by competitors. Thirdly, the objectives may have been achieved at the opportunity cost of not doing other things which needed to be done and which could have made a greater contribution to the organisation. This last point might be considered a failing of the objective-setting exercise, as it has set as objectives things which are not really important. But objective setting is not easy and the objectives which are set are often flawed. Furthermore, it can be extremely difficult to anticipate, at appraisal time, developmental opportunities which might arise during the period before the next appraisal. I would suggest that it is extremely dangerous to allow appraisees to form the opinion that 'All I've got to do to perform well is to meet this set of objectives.'

These points can be inverted to answer the question whether failure to meet objectives equates with poor performance. Also, it should be noted that while an objective may not be achieved, progress towards an objective may make a significant contribution. Take, for instance, the situation in which someone has an objective of reducing operating costs by 10 per cent while maintaining current service levels. If they manage only an 8 per cent reduction this is, strictly speaking, a failure, but surely it is a better performance than merely reducing operating costs by 3 per cent? A simplistic pass/fail approach can't be taken towards assessing the achievement of objectives. Finally, any overall assessment must also look at what has been achieved over and above the objectives set. Be wary of taking a blinkered or mechanistic approach.

Identifying training needs – a competency approach

This chapter presents a model, based on a specific example, of how to analyse training needs and is based on a 'competency' approach. A competency approach means identifying the competencies required to meet the duties of the job and then using them to analyse the individual's actual performance and training needs.

Rather than working from a generic list of skills, the starting point should be the job itself as outlined in the job description. From this you should proceed to identify the skills required to fulfil effectively each element of the job. As you do so, you need to reflect on the experience you have of the appraisee performing these skills. This process involves 'critical incidence' review, a process by which the appraiser seeks to recall particular incidents which illustrate the appraisee doing this aspect of their job well, adequately or not so well. In the process of critical incident review, it's important to remember to review incidents from the whole of the appraisal period and not just recent events which may be foremost in your memory.

As you analyse each element in the job description, the skills required and the appraisee's aptitude, ask yourself a series of key questions which will help you to examine your real feelings about the appraisee's performance. These questions are of two types: 'Does he/she ...?' and 'Would I trust him/her to ...?'

The example which follows illustrates the processes. It's based on a marketing job, that of assistant product manager in a plastic tubes manufacturing business. As you look at this example, think about how you could apply this technique to the jobs you have to appraise. You might also ask yourself whether the job descriptions you have for your staff provide an appropriate level of detail and are up to date.

Through this process you can be much more specific in identifying the training needs of the individual appraisee. By being more specific in this way you can also ensure that training is more specifically targeted. For instance, instead of blandly identifying that Jayne needs to develop her communication skills, her manager should be able to pinpoint that she needs help in participating in team meetings and particularly in sticking to the point, listening to others' ideas and supporting rather than squashing the contribution of others. When needs are identified as specifically as this, appropriate action can be taken and much unnecessary training can be avoided. Jayne probably doesn't need a course on 'communication' skills or even 'meeting' skills. What she probably needs is a quiet word in her ear from her line manager to make her think about her conduct in meetings.

Contributing to, in conjunction with the Product Manager and Marketing Assistant, the planning and introduction of new brochures and other promotional items, eg advertising, labels, fitting instructions, direct mail, giveaways . . .

Thinking skills
Does she:

- originate ideas;
- make useful suggestions building on others' ideas;
- unreasonably criticise others' ideas;
- recognise need for commercial realism?

Figure 8.1 *An example of the key-questions technique*

Interpersonal/discussing skills
Does she:

- have a co-operative working relationship with colleagues;
- participate constructively in group discussion?

Organising skills
Does she:

- produce proper project plans;
- monitor progress against plans and report on variance;
- meet deadlines without panic;
- produce material to desired standard and without errors in detail?

Supporting the Marketing Assistant with exhibitions, roadshows and promotional events for distributors and customers . . .

Organising skills
Does she:

- produce elements required on time and to spec?

Selling skills
Does she:

- present herself well on an exhibition stand;
- hold back from making contact with visitors;
- get too involved in discussions with customers;
- have a clear idea of, and stick to, selling objectives on the stand?

Would I trust her to man the stand alone for a long period?

Initiating, researching and writing press releases for trade journals, local press and *ad hoc* articles in conjunction with the Marketing Assistant.

Writing skills
Does she:

- write in a style appropriate for press releases and *ad hoc* articles;
- get an acceptable number of press releases published and in the right journals;
- circulate press releases widely and to the right journals?

Would I trust her to write a release without vetting it myself?
Do I make many changes to the writing she produces?

---

2   *Assisting with the review of sales and profitability*
Planning, constructing and printing of price lists . . .

Organising skills
Does she:
* produce accurate price lists on time?

Assisting with the recommendation and setting of price and
discount levels for existing and new products . . .

Pricing skills
Does she:
* know enough about what our competitors are charging;
* understand the basis of costing, contribution and margins;
* understand about price elasticity?

Regular analysis of company statistics, primarily for the monthly
market report.

Numerical/analytical skills
Does she:
* present detailed figures without analysis;
* use visuals well to present figures in a meaningful way;
* recognise which performance measures are relevant;
* make proper use of comparative figures;
* produce reports which are short and to the point?

Would I be happy to submit her reports to a higher level without
making any changes myself?

Figure 8.1   *An example of the key-questions technique*

9 Preparing for the appraisal discussion

The appraisal 'interview' or 'discussion' lies at the heart of most appraisal systems. Leading these discussions can be a daunting and emotionally-charged activity. As in all forms of communication, appraisal benefits greatly from time invested in preparation. As an appraiser your responsibility is not only to prepare yourself for this interaction, but also to help the appraisee to prepare.

Gathering information

The first stage in preparation has to be the gathering and collating of the information on which the appraisal is to be based. As we recognised in Chapter 3, appraisal should be an ongoing process. This means not only that the line-manager should be constantly providing feedback to the appraisee, but also that the line-manager should be constantly monitoring the appraisee's performance and gathering information relevant to the formal appraisal.

Part of this process may involve critical incident review. I have already referred in Chapter 8 to the value of this technique in analysing performance and identifying training needs. As I remarked then, one of the problems which impedes the objectivity of appraisal is the tendency of appraisers to allow recent events to colour their view of the whole period under review. To avoid this distortion you might find it helpful to make a note of critical incidents (specific instances of good or poor performance to illustrate a specific point) throughout the review period.

If you have a point you want to make about an appraisee's behaviour, then you need to be well prepared with the facts and be able to use them to illustrate your point. Again, this will involve gathering information by looking for the facts to test out a specific hypothesis. For instance, you may feel that your secretary's typing standards are not as good as they should be, or that they have dropped recently. If you wish to discuss this matter with her, you can't merely say: 'I'm not very happy with your typing standards lately.' You need some measure of what those standards actually are. One way of obtaining this would be to do a log over a week or so, noting the average number of avoidable mistakes occurring per A4 page. This would provide the concrete evidence on which to base your discussion with her.

Be careful not to fall into the trap of collecting information merely to support your impressions. In assessing someone's performance you need to formulate and test hypotheses. Don't look just for information/incidents that support your hypothesis – look also for information/incidents which contradict it.

Often the information you need is not just that based on your first-hand experience of the appraisee's performance. You need to explore how well he/she has performed for other managers and departments which he/she may be responsible for servicing. This will be particularly important if you are operating a matrix management system.

The problem that often occurs with matrix management is that the line-manager feels that he/she no longer has control over, or responsibility for, individual staff members. This misinterpretation of matrix management can mean that the management of some individuals falls between two stools and that they actually receive no proper management at all.

The key to success in matrix management is to see yourself as heading a team of specialists providing services to clients. Your clients are the managers of the various projects on which your specialists are engaged. Your clients may be external or internal. Constant monitoring of client satisfaction and exploration of opportunities to enhance the quality of service provided then become central features of your role as line manager.

This monitoring process also includes providing feedback to your staff. This should be done on a regular basis, but it also forms part of formal appraisal. Thus an essential part of your preparation for appraisal will be gathering information from your 'clients' on the performance of your appraisees.

Once you have gathered the information, you have to decide which aspects of performance to focus on and which information you feel is pertinent. You will also need to think about how the discussion might be structured to bring in the various points you want to raise. These are matters to which we will return in later chapters.

Preparing the appraisee

If you are to have a two-way discussion with an appraisee, it's just as important for the appraisee to be prepared as it is for you. Not only should the appraisee have some idea of the issues which he/she wants to raise, the appraisee should also be equipped to discuss the points you want to raise. Unfortunately, too often appraisees see their roles as either passive or defensive. You need to encourage your staff to be proactive, taking some initiative towards ensuring the effectiveness of the discussion and the value of the appraisal process.

You also need to ensure that they are familiar with the way the appraisal system works, its purpose and their rights and responsibilities under it. This process should be part of the induction of every new member of staff, and if this has not been the case in the past, it should be a subject for team briefing. It is not good enough to tell someone for the first time how the appraisal system works just as the appraisal round is due.

Reference was made in Chapter 4 to the value of pre-appraisal forms. If your system does not include this process and you don't feel you can adopt it, you might find it a useful alternative to send the appraisee a briefing memo. This briefing might act both as a reminder as to how the system is supposed to operate and as an outline agenda – at least specifying some of the topics you want to raise. However, it shouldn't be seen as a fixed agenda – it will be suggested later that building a detailed agenda together is a valuable way of starting the discussion (see Chapter 11).

Figure 9.1 presents an example of a briefing note. You might like to use it as a model to prepare one of your own. The more you can personalise it, the more effective it will be – try to make it appear different from other pieces of appraisal 'bumph' produced by Personnel. Amend and extend the note to suit your own style and circumstances and the workings of your own appraisal system. Even if formal notification of the appraisal round is provided by the personnel department, it's still worthwhile adding your own personal note.

MEMORANDUM

To: John Smith
From: Jayne White
Date: 6 September
Subject: ANNUAL APPRAISAL

We have agreed to meet for your annual appraisal discussion at 2.30 on Monday 20 September. To help us both get the best from the discussion it would be useful if you would give some prior consideration to any topics you would like to talk about.

Appraisal provides you with the opportunity to:
● receive feedback on your performance;
● have your achievements recognised;
● raise performance issues which are of concern to you;
● explore actions to improve performance and maximise your contribution.

Please take a little time to re-familiarise yourself with the appraisal system and your rights and responsibilities under it.

Remember the overall purpose is to help you perform – not only increasing your contribution to the department, but also enhancing your job satisfaction and career development prospects.

Figure 9.1   *Example of a briefing memo*

Preparing the environment

All face-to-face communications are affected by the physical environment in which they take place. Environmental considerations encompass furnishing and seating arrangements, lighting, noise and distractions. For an appraisal discussion to be effective, take as much control as you can over environmental factors.

The first issue to decide is where the discussion should take place. It should be confidential, therefore, if you are in an open plan or shared office you will have to find somewhere else to hold it. Even if you do have an office of your own there are advantages in booking a meeting room. This is neutral territory and choosing such territory may create a greater sense of equality and joint ownership.

Seating arrangements will also affect the extent to which the appraisee feels this sense of joint ownership. Depending on your circumstances, you may be able to exercise some valuable choice over the way the room is arranged and where you sit. Broadly these choices range through those illustrated in Figure 9.2.

Arrangement 1

This layout creates a very formal atmosphere. The desk acts as a barrier to communication and emphasises the 'distance' between appraiser and appraisee. Although this may diminish the sense of joint ownership and equality, it is not necessarily detrimental to the appraisal discussion. The 'distance' might be appropriate to your management style and both you and the appraisee might feel more comfortable with the degree of protection it provides. However, you need to be aware of the implications of this layout so that you use it only when you have no choice or when you do so as a conscious act. If you have to conduct the appraisal discussion across your desk, tidy up first – messy desks show a lack of preparation and the clutter itself acts as a barrier.

Arrangement 2

This layout does away with the barrier, but may leave the appraisee feeling exposed and vulnerable. He/she will feel

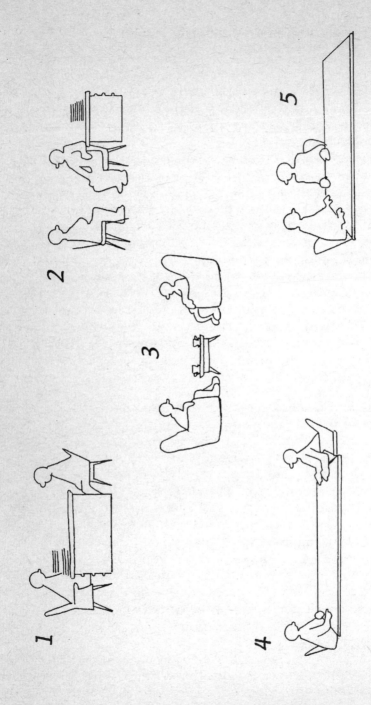

Figure 9.2 The communicating environment

further disadvantaged as you may be the only one with somewhere to rest your papers (and your elbows).

Arrangement 3

Low comfortable chairs around the coffee table is an option that appeals to many managers, as it creates a relaxed informal atmosphere. However, this may be _too_ informal for the appraisal process. This arrangement also presents problems if either party needs to refer to papers, or wants to make notes.

Remember that the appraisal discussion needs to be businesslike and is not just a cosy chat. I was told of a manager who believed that the appraisal 'interview' should be a 'relaxed and informal' affair and so conducted sessions at the pub. One problem was that by the end of the discussion both parties were often as 'relaxed and informal as newts'!

Arrangements 4 and 5

The best option is for appraiser and appraisee to sit at a table in a meeting room. The table allows both parties to have papers in front of them and it is also more 'neutral' territory than using the appraiser's desk.

Appraisee and appraiser should sit fairly close to each other but not so close that they invade each other's 'personal space'. Sitting directly facing each other may create a confrontational atmosphere. Sitting next to each other produces a more collaborative atmosphere. With an oblong table it works best if the appraiser sits at the short side and the appraisee sits at right angles close to him/her on the long side. At round tables appraiser and appraisee should also sit close to each other rather than diametrically opposite.

Other factors

You also need to take account of factors such as lighting. Don't sit with the light behind you shining directly into the appraisee's eyes!

Control extraneous noise. If the builders are in the process of knocking down the wall of the adjoining office, get them to stop or otherwise rearrange the time or place of the meeting.

Don't be tempted to battle on in spite of the noise – noise not only distracts, it also creates feelings of hostility. Good preparation means anticipating and avoiding these sorts of problems.

Lastly, in preparing the environment, ensure you preclude all interruptions. Controlling interruptions is particularly important if you are using your own office. During the time that you've set aside for the appraisal discussion it is very unlikely that there is anything sufficiently urgent to take precedence and justify an interruption. This is an issue of priorities. Allowing interruptions not only disrupts the discussion, it gives appraisees the message that you regard them and the appraisal as comparatively unimportant. During the allotted time the most important issue is appraisal and the most important person is the appraisee – not your managing director or even a significant client.

Remember to divert your telephone. Posting a 'do not disturb' sign on the door might also help, but more effective control of interruptions involves telling potential interrupters about when you will be available, not just telling them that you're not.

10 Communicating and listening

Leading an appraisal discussion requires good face-to-face communication skills. The onus on having those skills may be considerable, particularly if you have to overcome an appraisee's lack of communication skill or a negative attitude.

We've already recognised that to be effective and worthwhile, the appraisal process needs to be shared and that it needs to create a sense of joint ownership. This means that communication has to be two-way and that you have to work at creating a genuine dialogue. This involves not only expressing yourself clearly and unambiguously, but also listening to what the appraisee has to say and checking both parties' understanding.

As a manager, you'll probably be well aware of many of the pitfalls that are associated with face-to-face communication. Nonetheless, it's worthwhile reminding yourself of them so that you can avoid the dangers of miscommunication undermining the effectiveness of the appraisal process.

Inappropriate language

The language you use has to be appropriate to your listener's level of understanding. Unfortunately we get into the habit of using certain words and don't ask ourselves often enough whether or not the person we're talking to understands them. This is particularly significant where there are differences in technical understanding between the two parties to a conversation. Clearly you need to choose your words carefully when discussing technical matters with non-specialists. This may not seem to be too much of a problem in an appraisal discussion – after all, both you and the appraisee are in the same business or profession. Be careful nonetheless that you don't overlook the dangers of 'management speak' – using language and referring to concepts which may be second nature when talking with your peers, but which may not be familiar to other staff.

You also need to be careful when using abbreviations and acronyms. It's easy to fall into the habit of using a set of initials while forgetting that this abbreviation may mean nothing to the other party. Sometimes, of course, a set of initials can mean more than one thing. One organisation used the abbreviation SDI to refer to its 'Staff Development Interview' scheme, while for one group of specialists covered by the scheme, those same letters meant 'Selective Dissemination of Information'.

It is not only technical language which causes difficulties. People often fail to understand each other because one of the parties to the conversation uses high-faluting words rather than colloquial, everyday words and phrases. A related danger is using foreign words and phrases – 'quid pro quo', 'mea culpa', 'laissez-faire', 'Zeitgeist', to list but a few examples. Be sensitive, therefore, to the social and educational background (not just the educational level) and vocabulary range of the person with whom you're dealing.

The problem is often compounded by a listener's unwillingness to admit that he/she is unfamiliar with a word, phrase, abbreviation or acronym. It's quite a normal reaction to 'let it go' and hope that the meaning can be deciphered from context as the conversation continues. Two important points follow. First, just because someone doesn't ask you to clarify or explain a term, don't assume that they've understood it. Secondly, if someone uses a phrase with which you're unfamiliar, be prepared to stop the conversation and ask for clarification. If you 'let it go' and then find you aren't able to unravel the meaning from the context, your ultimate embarrassment will be all the greater.

Another language problem is that people are sometimes over ambitious with the words they use and thus use them incorrectly. It's one thing to understand fairly well in a passive sense what a word means; it's another to use it correctly in an active manner. This is not only a warning that we have to be careful about the words we use, but also a reminder that confusion may stem from the other party using words in the wrong context. If what the other party says seems odd, then question him/her about the use of a particular word. Sometimes as a result of some temporary aberration people use words in a way which they don't intend – sometimes saying the exact opposite of what they mean! Again, the point is not to let yourself get confused and not to assume the speaker necessarily means what he/she is saying. If the message you're getting isn't clear or doesn't make sense, check out your understanding with the other party.

Hidden messages

While we need to be careful about how the language we use impacts upon the explicit messages we give and receive, we need also to recognise that much of our communication takes place not on an explicit level but as a series of hidden messages or signals from which it is expected the listener will draw the correct inference. Here are some examples. 'You're often late for meetings. This mustn't continue and you must get there on time' may be expressed as 'We must try to start our meetings more punctually'. 'Stop doing it that way' becomes 'I'd rather you found another way of doing it'. 'I wouldn't normally consider such an offer' may actually mean 'Please vary your terms so that I can consider this offer'. 'It would be very difficult' doesn't necessarily mean the same as 'It's impossible'; it may mean 'You'll have to work harder to persuade me and make it more worth my while'.

Communicating involves both giving, and picking up on, hidden messages. It is a process which can be fraught with danger as the intended inference may not be drawn. The listener may simply assume you mean what you say. At the same time if you fail to pick up the signals from the other party, you may miss the opportunity to explore important avenues of discussion.

Using indirect language requires a mutual understanding of the rules of the game. An indirect message is particularly characteristic of the way the English middle-class use language, but people from other cultures may adopt a more direct approach. Although this may be less ambiguous in meaning, it can upset you if you are not used to making your messages explicit. Be careful not to overreact.

Audibility difficulties

Problems of hearing clearly what the other person is saying, and of being heard yourself, can have a detrimental impact upon the communication process. A number of factors affect audibility – hearing or speech impediments, accents, speaking too quietly, speaking too fast or too slowly or monotonously, putting a hand in front of the mouth or looking in the wrong direction while speaking, and extraneous background noises. Audibility difficulties create tension and awkwardness. Clearly you've got to be careful to speak as audibly as you can. If you can't hear or decipher what an appraisee is saying, you've got to be prepared to admit it and ask him/her to speak louder, more slowly or whatever. Avoid the temptation we referred to above of 'letting it go' in the hope that you'll be able to work out what was said later.

The implications of tone

A speaker's tone contributes considerably to the meaning projected and the inferences taken in any communication. Tone may be considered both in its literal sense, as the pitch of the voice, and in the more literary sense as the style or choice of phrasing.

Pitch

As you will be aware, the tone of voice (pitch) may be used to convey a meaning contrary to the actual words used. This is particularly so when sarcastic comments are made. Even in platonic circumstances, the phrase 'I love you' can be one of appreciation or complaint depending upon the tone employed. While we derive much of our understanding from vocal tone, we must be careful not to read too much into it or draw the wrong inference. A comment which sounds sarcastic may not be intended as such. Be careful not to overreact to a tone which you interpret as sarcastic (even if that is clearly its intent). Your reaction may lead to a cycle of hostility and defensiveness.

Phrasing

When we look at the second meaning of tone, the style or phrasing, again it is often the way that people react to the tone which determines how the communication proceeds. In a fascinating study, management psychologist Peter Honey* shows how people respond differently depending upon whether an idea is expressed as a 'suggestion' or as a 'proposal'. His study shows that what he calls 'suggesting behaviour' (suggesting a possible course of action in a question form – 'shall we do so and so?; 'how about doing so and so?') is far more likely to produce a positive 'supporting' response ('that's a good idea'; 'that would certainly help') than is the case when 'proposing behaviour' is used. 'Proposing behaviour' involves proposing a possible course of action in the form of a statement, announcement or instruction – 'we will do so and so'; 'I suggest you do so and so'; 'let's do so and so'; 'I propose we do so and so'. While 'suggesting behaviour' tends to produce 'supporting behaviour', 'proposing behaviour' most commonly produces 'difficulty stating' by way of response. Honey's conclusion is simple: if you want to get people's support you're more likely to succeed when you phrase an idea as a suggestion rather than as a proposition. Clearly this can be critical in ensuring effective communication during an appraisal discussion.

Contradiction of words and gestures

Just as tone can be at variance with the words used, so body language can convey a contradictory message. For instance, your appraisee may say 'Yes, I agree, I'll do that', but the body stance may be saying 'No, I don't want to do that'.

Watch out for defensive or negative gestures. These involve a combination of gestures which may include a glum facial

_____

* Peter Honey, *Face to Face*, Gower, 1988.

expression, avoidance of eye contact, tightly folded arms and crossed legs. (Be careful not to read too much into a single gesture – it's a cluster of gestures that counts.) The appraisee who adopts these gestures but says he agrees, is in fact suggesting that he does not agree. Respond by picking up this message. 'I get the feeling you may not be too happy about this. Can we discuss it a little further?'

One of the problems with defensive body language is that it's contagious. On seeing someone behave in a defensive way, it's very easy to respond subconsciously by adopting the same 'tight' gestures. The result can be a cycle of defensiveness and even hostility. The antidote to defensive/negative gestures is to adopt open and positive gestures – such as unfolding arms and legs. This may be almost painful at first (as it makes you feel more exposed and vulnerable), but its effect is to slowly diffuse tensions and break down some of the barriers.

Lack of structure

Unstructured, rambling conversations are difficult to follow. It's all too easy to get distracted and fail to stick to the point. Quick-thinking intelligent minds may be particularly prone to going off at a tangent. Good communication requires that conversations be kept focused and well structured.

You need to have a good idea of what you want to say. Avoid getting yourself distracted and if you do, you need to be able to take explicit action to pull the conversation back on course: 'Now, the point we were discussing was ...' or 'Now, let's get back to the main point of the discussion', or 'Okay, where were we? What we need to decide is how we're going to ...'.

Your ability to stay on target, or to get back on course should the conversation stray, is greatly aided by having an agreed agenda. A good appraisal (or indeed any two-way discussion) will involve agreeing an agenda and using summaries to maintain control. This important point is picked up in Chapter 11 which examines the process of structuring the appraisal discussion.

Assumptions and prejudices

One of the main pitfalls in face-to-face communication is failing to listen properly. All too often what we hear is what we expect to hear, rather than what is actually being said. Communication is impaired by the assumptions or prejudgements we make about the other party. Once we have formed a view of someone or their position, it can be very difficult for us to rid ourselves of the preconception and evaluate objectively what he/she is actually saying. A typical pitfall is to form the prejudice that 'Fred' is an awkward character. When appraising 'Fred' the danger is that we interpret whatever he says as further evidence of his awkwardness rather than listening carefully and evaluating what he is actually saying. 'Fred' might actually be making some quite constructive comments, but as we don't expect 'Fred' to be constructive we might dismiss what he has to say out of hand.

Effective listening

From the above discussion it follows that good communication requires good listening skills. It's important to recognise that listening is not a passive process, but rather requires conscious effort and participation. This mnemonic may help you think about the requirements of effective listening.

L = Look interested
I = Involve yourself by questioning
S = Stay on target
T = Test your understanding
E = Evaluate the message
N = Neutralise your feelings

Look interested means adopting a positive and encouraging body language – leaning forward slightly, nodding in recognition of what's being said and even adding the odd 'aha'.

Involve yourself by questioning means using questions to maintain interest and involvement and choosing your questions to show the appraisee you're following the logic of what he/she is saying.

Stay on target means intervening carefully to draw the appraisee back on course, or asking him/her to make clear the relevance of what he/she is saying to the topic under discussion.

Test your understanding involves intervening to summarise in your own words what's been said: 'Now let me see if I've got this right. What you're saying is ...'.

Evaluate the message involves the mental processing of the message, relating it to what you already know or to your own position and assessing the implications.

Neutralise your feelings means being conscious of your prejudices and assumptions and working actively to prevent them impairing the listening process.

11 *Structuring the appraisal discussion*

To be effective, appraisal meetings require structure. Structure gives the appraisee a sense of direction, provides you with a means of controlling the discussion and helps to ensure that all relevant issues are covered.

A well-structured appraisal discussion will have three discrete phases: a beginning, a middle and an end.

Beginnings

It's vitally important to get off to the right start by establishing a relaxed but positive atmosphere. It's worthwhile, therefore, spending a little time thinking about how you're going to kick off. The 'beginning' phase has three elements:

- a 'chat-gap';
- a review of the purpose of the meeting;
- a building of the agenda.

Chat-gap

The chat-gap is a few words of social discussion before the real business begins and is part and parcel of the social niceties of doing business in most cultures. A short chat-gap is a useful way of relaxing the appraisee. It's important that the chat-gap shouldn't appear too contrived and, of course, that it should be carefully controlled so that the appraisee isn't led off into a lengthy discussion unrelated to the purpose of the meeting.

Here are two examples which might be appropriate:

> **Appraiser**: Ah, Jane come in and take a seat. How are things with you?
>
> **Jane**: Not too bad.
>
> **Apprasier**: How's John getting on these days – still keen on his football?
>
> **Jane**: Yes – he's playing for the School Under-13's.
>
> **Appraiser**: Good. I used to enjoy football when I was at school. I hope he keeps up his interest. Now, as you know we're here today for your annual appraisal discussion… .

In this example the chat-gap is kept short and, although almost ritualistic, is personalised. The appraising manager is showing that he takes a personal interest in the appraisee and remembers the name of her son and his interest in football. The appraiser is recognising the individuality of the appraisee.

The second example uses the chat-gap to create a positive atmosphere by introducing a few words of appreciation related to a job in hand.

> **Appraiser**: Come in, Penny. Take a seat. Just before we begin I thought you might like to know Jill's just been on the phone. She was very impressed by your designs for Martland and thinks we'll be able to win this one. Well done.
> Now let's get down to business. As you know we're here …

In both these examples the end of the chat-gap is clearly signalled. This is important otherwise the formal discussion may get under way without either party being aware that it has begun and without some of the other preliminaries of the 'beginning phase' being dealt with.

Review of meeting's purpose

The next step is to review briefly the purpose of the meeting. Something along the following lines might be appropriate:

> **Appraiser**: Now as you know, we're here for your annual appraisal interview. The purpose of the interview is to look at how your job's been going over the last year (what's gone well and what hasn't gone so well); to look at anything we can do to help you do your job better, or enjoy it more; to look at any opportunities you feel there might be to make even greater use of your talents; and, of course, to look at the future.

This may also be a good time to refer to note making: 'I shall be making some notes throughout, and at the end of our discussion I'd like you to summarise any action we agree, so you might like to make some notes as well.'

Building the agenda

Having made a brief statement of the purpose of the meeting you are now in a position to move on to the agenda building phase. It is essential to ensure that you share the process of agenda building and that you don't simply impose your own.
  Following from the previous example you could initiate the agenda-building phase in the following way:

> **Appraiser**: Now, I've got one or two items I particularly want to discuss and I'm sure you've also got some. So why don't we start by mapping out an agenda together. All right?

Ninety-nine per cent of the time the appraisee will say 'Okay' or 'Fine'. By asking appraisees for their assent in this way you are recognising their rights to be consulted over how the meeting is conducted and emphasising the joint-ownership of the process.

The discussion may continue:

> **Appraiser**: The main points I want to look at are: the use of the computer, the issue of workloads and deadlines; and relation-ships with other members of the team. Now what do you want to tackle?
>
> **Appraisee**: Well, I want to talk about the equipment prob-lems, and the need for more staff.
>
> **Appraiser**: Okay then. These seem to go together quite well. Let's start off by talking about equipment problems in general and bring in there the use of the computer. Second we can tackle the issue of workloads and deadlines, and that will no doubt involve us in looking at the issue of staff levels. And then we can move on to look at relationships with the rest of the team. But before getting into these detailed points I'd like us to start off by taking an overview of the period as a whole and what we've achieved. Is that all right?

The appraiser might continue:

> **Appraiser**: How do you think things have gone over the last 12 months?

Again, the appraisee's assent is sought and will nearly always be given. You might then ask an open question to get the appraisee talking further.

> **Appraiser**: I think it would make sense if we follow the format of the appraisal form and for us to focus on each of the desig-nated performance areas in turn – looking at what's gone well, addressing any problems and deciding any action we need to take to help you perform in the future. We can then look at your overall performance rating and promotion prospects. Is that okay?

This question will probably be enough to get the appraisee to open up but some might be a bit reluctant and answer 'Fine' or 'Not too bad', in which case some form of probing or follow-up question will be needed. This might be 'What do you think the main achievements have been ...?'

The point here is that you should aim to get the appraisee talking early, and use appropriate questions to get the conversation going. Questioning technique is looked at in further detail in Chapter 12.

An alternative agenda may be provided by the appraisal form. After outlining the purpose of the appraisal discussion you might like to proceed:

> **Appraiser**: We need a structure for our discussion. Why don't we follow the form and use that as our framework? Hopefully, that'll allow us to cover all the important issues. If there's anything you think we might miss, please don't hesitate to say so. Is that okay?

Here there has been less involvement of the appraisee in building the agenda. However, the structure of the agenda is neutral in so far as it has been imposed not by the appraiser, but by the system itself. Again the appraiser asks for, and will get, the appraisee's assent.

Another structure might be one provided by a job description. After outlining the purpose of the interview, you could proceed by saying:

> **Appraiser**: I'm very keen we cover every aspect of the job. How about structuring our discussion around the job description, looking at each item in turn? Then we can look at any other points we want to discuss. Is there anything in particular you'd like to flag up at this stage?

This approach requires an up-to-date and realistic job description. It also requires that the appraisee's attention has been drawn to the job description as part of their preparation.

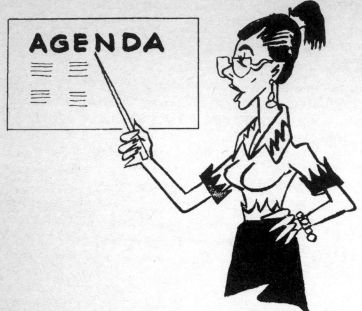

'Now this is the agenda you're going to agree to follow.'

Middles

The 'middle' or main part of the meeting is going to be taken up by each of the agenda items. Each item itself needs to be approached in a structured way with a clear indication of the start of the point which is being discussed and a summary at the end confirming agreed action and signalling that that item has now been dealt with. You need to be careful that discussion doesn't wander off the point and be prepared to say things like, 'I think that's a very important point, but it's really best if we leave it until we come onto the next item on the agenda. What we've got to do is concentrate on ... and agree how we're going to tackle it.'

   Don't move on to the next item until you've agreed specific action on the point under discussion. It's always useful to ask yourself 'Have we agreed who is going to do what by when?' Use the agenda to control the discussion, preventing the appraisee jumping ahead or going back over old ground and discipline yourself to follow the same rules.

Endings

As with 'beginnings', endings can be subdivided into three elements. These are:

- signalling the end;
- summarising actions;
- concluding.

Signalling the end

The end of the meeting needs to be clearly signalled. However, before moving into the last phase, you must check that there are no additional matters the appraisee wants to raise. You might try the following formula: 'Okay, we've covered all the agenda items. I want to move on now to the conclusion, but before we do so, can I check – are there any additional issues you want to raise?' If you don't check in this way one of two things may happen. Either you miss the opportunity to explore an issue of concern to the appraisee, or the appraisee may intervene and disrupt the closing procedure.

Summarising actions

Once you've gained agreement to move on to the end, the next stage should be to summarise the actions discussed and agreed throughout the meeting.

It can be useful to ask the appraisee to do the summary. 'Okay. We've discussed a lot of issues this afternoon. I think it would help both of us if you would summarise the main points and the action we've agreed.'

This acts as a useful check. It may help you realise that you haven't put over a point as well as you wanted and that you need to clarify it a little further. It also provides a means of testing if the appraisee has really internalised the action agreed. Appraisees may miss out or skate over something they are not really happy about or they may indicate reluctance or unhappiness by tone or body language. As an appraiser you need to be able to pick up these signals and tackle the issue with sensitivity. For instance, 'You didn't mention the .... Is there anything you're not happy about?' or 'I get the feeling that you're not entirely happy about .... Are there some difficulties about doing it which we haven't discussed fully?'

Concluding

Close the discussion with a one or two line summary yourself and leave the meeting on a high note, thanking the appraisee for his/her participation.

Appraiser: Well we've had our difficulties in the past, but if we both work on implementing the points we discussed this afternoon, I think we'll be able to work much better in the future. Thanks very much for your time and cooperation.

Or: Let me just say again how pleased I am with your overall performance. Keep up the good work and thank you for all your helpful comments this afternoon.

---

12 *Questioning technique*

Asking questions is an essential part of leading the discussion. Questions are necessary to find out information and to explore attitudes. As an appraiser, it's useful to think of yourself as a detective. You have some of the evidence, but you need to find out more to get a fuller picture from the appraisee. You have some leads, but you need to check them out. The way in which you uncover the evidence and check out the value of the leads is by asking questions and probing to get the information you require. Questions are also a vital means of getting the appraisee to talk – involving him/her in the discussion and avoiding the dangers of monologue. They are also a way of getting the appraisee to reflect – giving consideration to alternative courses of action and developing their own insights.

This brief chapter provides an analysis of the range of question types available and the situations in which particular question types are most suitable.

Questions are usually divided into two broad categories: 'closed' and 'open'. Closed questions are those which may produce a specific response, such as 'Yes', 'No', or '272'. Open questions, on the other hand, require more elaborate and open-ended answers. Examples of **closed** questions include:

- 'How many of your staff left during the last 12 months?'
- 'Do you enjoy this aspect of your work?'
- 'Does this happen often?'

Examples of **open** questions include:

- 'What are the reasons for the level of staff turnover?'
- 'Which aspects of your job do you enjoy most?'
- 'Why does this happen so often?'

Open questions may also take the form of inviting the interviewee to talk:

● 'Tell me about the problem with Mandy.'

Open and closed questions need to be used in combination: open questions to develop discussion and look at some of the reasons for certain things; closed questions to uncover specific facts and attitudes.

There are, of course, various types of open and closed questions and a variety of ways of classifying question format. Figure 12.1 shows some of the types of question you might consider employing together with some comments on their usefulness.

Probing (open)
Exactly what happened next?
For obtaining additional detail and getting the appraise to be specific.

Probing (closed)
How old were you then?
For establishing specific points and probing single facts.

Reflective
You feel upset about the move?
(Repeats verbatim the emotional content of an appraisee's statement.) To show interest and to help the appraisee discuss difficult issues.

Leading
I suppose you're sorry now, are you?
Leads the appraisee towards a predetermined answer. Can be useful for gaining verbal agreement to a viewpoint, but may not lead to commitment.

Hypothetical
What would you do if ...?
(Question based on a hypothetical situation in the future.)

Useful in getting the appraisee to think about new areas or additional dimensions to an issue. Not useful if the hypothetical situation can be seen as very unlikely to occur.

Multiple
A string of questions without allowing the appraisee time to answer each one in turn. This technique may be useful in Nazi-style interrogation. It is not appropriate in appraisal.

Comparison
Would you prefer advancement on the managerial or the technical side?
Useful to help the appraisee focus attention on choices, but not useful if the choices are unrealistic.

Figure 12.1 *Question formats*

Be careful to choose the appropriate question type and to phrase your question in the right way. Appraisers find it all too easy to express themselves in a way which is emotionally charged or prejudicial with the result that they produce negative or defensive responses to their questions. For instance, instead of 'Was it time pressure or cost that governed your decision?' (a phrasing which directs the appraisee to a choice of only two answers), it might be better to ask the more open question 'What factors did you consider in making your decision?'

An important part of questioning technique is listening for the answers. This involves ensuring that questions and statements are not phrased so as to involve a presupposition as to the answer. For instance, 'I suppose you did it that way because ...?' is really a way of answering the question for the appraisee. It might be more appropriate to ask the open question 'Why did you do it that way?' Secondly, it's important to give the appraisee time to answer the question. Don't be worried if the appraisee pauses for a while before answering. The pause may simply be an indication that the appraisee is thinking about how to answer, not that he/she has no answer to give at all. Above all, avoid being overwilling to jump in and fill in the silence. Too often appraisers are tempted into answering their own questions or into following up one unanswered question with another.

Recently I observed an amusing example of inappropriate questioning technique during an appraisal role-play exercise. A manager, who was also a solicitor, slipped comfortably into his natural style, premising nearly every question with the phrase 'You would agree, would you not ...?' The tone, clearly reminiscent of a courtroom cross-examination, produced a wry smile from his role-play partner and the response: 'I refuse to take part in this appraisal discussion on the grounds that I may be required to incriminate myself!'

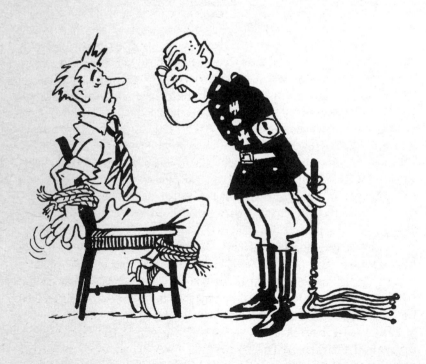

'We have ways of making you talk.'

13 | *Constructive criticism*

I suggested in Chapter 3 that one of the reasons why many managers feel uncomfortable with appraisal is that they don't like criticising their staff. Such fears are not unwarranted. Even with an appraisee whose performance is good, discussing the scope to improve performance may imply some form of criticism. With those whose performance falls below expected standards, there is likely to be a highly critical content within the appraisal discussion. Appraisers often fear that they will handle criticising badly, thus undermining the appraisee's confidence or motivation and creating resentment. A related fear is that by being critical, an appraiser may make him/herself vulnerable to counter-criticism from the appraisee. As well as being ill-equipped to give criticism, appraisers may be ill-equipped to receive it.

You might be tempted to avoid the risk of conflict and skate around the difficult areas. As a result there can be a paradox where the most 'difficult' appraisee receives the least critical appraisal and the best performing appraisee may receive a disproportionate amount of criticism.

Fear of conflict should not lead you into ducking your responsibility to provide staff with critical feedback. If you do duck out, then poor standards of performance may continue and opportunities for improvement may be missed. You have a right to criticise your staff and, while you need to criticise skilfully and sensitively, there will be times when you have to face up to difficult situations.

While our concern here is with giving criticism in an appraisal situation, the skills are also applicable to other occasions. I have already made the point that criticism should not be reserved for the appraisal meeting. The formality of the process, which can sometimes be seen as affording some protection against 'personal awkwardness', may tempt you to store up criticisms for the occasion. This is bad appraisal, bad management and bad criticism. It's bad appraisal because the appraisal discussion should not contain any real surprises. It's bad management because critical feedback needs to be provided on a day-to-day basis. It is bad criticism because repressed criticism can lead to a build up of resentment which may find expression in some form of overreaction.

It's often said that as part of day-to-day management good managers should look for opportunities to praise their staff, showing that they notice what they do well and giving what are sometimes called 'positive strokes'. More contentiously it might be argued that good managers should look for opportunities to criticise their staff, showing that they notice what they do less well. On this basis managers get more used to, and skilled in, criticising, while staff get more used to a relationship in which they expect to be criticised and become more used to handling it. This is not to say that the manager/staff relationship should be one which is primarily based on criticism or that the primary aim of the manager should be to catch staff out. A relationship which encompasses criticism should be based also on acknowledging things that are done well. Praise and criticism need to be offered in balance. Praise buys the manager the leeway to criticise and the right to expect fair criticism to be taken fairly.

Criticism, of course, has to be constructive, that is to say directed towards changing things for the better. Criticising people without this aim is destructive, 'bitchy' and cannot be justified as part of a manager's rights and responsibilities.

Collect the evidence and test hypotheses

Collecting evidence is part of preparing for appraisal. Criticism needs to be specific and based on facts rather than impressions or feelings. Criticising someone for their time-keeping by saying, 'You seem to be coming in late a lot recently', necessarily leads to the rejoinder, 'When was I late?' Unless you have the specific evidence to back up the accusation you can be left floundering. Therefore you must make sure you have a full grasp of the pertinent facts before you raise such an issue.

As we said in Chapter 9, look for evidence to substantiate your criticisms. If you have a feeling that someone's performance is not what it should be in a particular area, check out that impression and see if the facts support it. You may actually find that your impressions cannot be substantiated and that your criticism would have been unfounded.

Ration the criticism

Even if there's a lot to criticise, you will have to ration your criticism for it to be effective. Choose the two or three most important points, or those which you think are most conducive to a solution. Minor points may have to be ignored. Be careful when dealing with appraisees who are good at receiving criticism. Because someone is skilled at taking criticism and apparently responsive, don't be tempted to 'pile it on'. Even people who are good at taking it will resent criticism if it becomes remorseless.

Avoid old ground

Don't use the appraisal meeting simply to repeat all the criticisms you've already made. If an issue has been dealt with and resolved, then it isn't pertinent to go over old ground. However, while the specifics of the issue may not be pertinent, it may well suggest a general point which may be worth exploring at a deeper level. One of the benefits of appraisal is that it allows you to take stock of a range of critical incidents and see if they reveal a pattern which in turn may allow you to identify fundamental performance issues.

Balance criticism and praise

I have already made the point that there needs to be a balance between criticism and praise within a working relationship. The need for balance applies also within a structured appraisal discussion. Look for the things you can praise to buy yourself the scope to raise the criticisms you want to. Even with a poor performer, if you actively look for something which is praiseworthy you can usually find it. The balance must be qualitative rather than merely quantitative. It's very easy to put together a few pat phrases of general praise and then follow them by detailed and specific criticism. I will make the point shortly that we need to be specific in our criticism. The point to remember here is that we need also to be specific in our praise.

Compartmentalise the criticism

If you have to criticise a particular aspect of an appraisee's performance, try to compartmentalise it so that you can move on to another, and hopefully happier, topic. Good use of an agenda as discussed in Chapter 11 makes this process easier. By moving through an agenda on a topic by topic basis, you can try to ensure that praise and criticism are distributed evenly throughout the discussion. This is preferable to a structure which has been called 'the criticism sandwich'. The 'criticism sandwich' starts with a slice of generalised praise, follows it with the criticism, and rounds off with a final slice of praise. Often the appraisee will listen to the praise with dread anticipation of the word 'but'. The need to distribute criticism and praise homogeneously throughout the discussion may quite reasonably be one of the factors which determines the order in which you wish to tackle the agenda.

Giving criticism

When we criticise, we need to encourage the recipient to respond positively. Avoid making personal attacks, try to defuse any aggression and build towards formulating joint solutions. A three-step approach is involved:

Step 1. Establish two-way communication about the problem.
Step 2. Focus on the specifics of the problem.
Step 3. Search for a joint solution to the problem.

Step 1 – Establish communication

It is essential to establish open communication and avoid

prompting an immediately negative, emotional, defensive response. Avoid personalising the issue and making extreme or absolute judgements. Adopt a neutral tone.

The example which follows shows four alternative ways of raising the same issue.

A Your presentations are appalling.

B I'm not happy with your presentations.

C We need to talk about your presentations.

D Er, um, I hope you don't mind, and it's only my opinion of course, and I could be wrong, but I was wondering whether you think there might be scope for you to improve your presentation.

A is highly confrontational – it expresses an opinion as though it were a fact. B is milder and at least recognises that the assessment relates to the personal opinion of the appraiser. C, however, is neutral yet direct. D is over-apologetic, non-assertive and counter-productive.

Step 2 – Focus on the specifics

If the person you're criticising responds in a negative or hostile way, let the wave of hostility ride over you. Don't get pulled into personal conflict. Ensure that you remain in control by moving on to discuss the specifics of the situation.

As I have already said, it is essential that you are prepared to discuss specifics and that you have the evidence to support the criticism you are making. Often the criticised's response will be to challenge you in terms of these specifics. You need to be able to respond, confident that you know what you're talking about.

If, as in the example above, you are criticising someone's presentations, it's not unlikely that they'll respond along the lines: 'What's wrong with my presentations?' If in turn you answer 'Well, they just don't seem to be going as well as they ought to be', this simply shows a lack of preparation on your part and misses the opportunity to focus on the real issues. It's vague and undermines the credibility of the criticism. Instead, a considered response along the lines of 'I'm concerned primarily with your use of the OHP. In last month's presentation I noticed ....' allows you to progress towards working out some solutions.

The example below presents another piece of dialogue with alternative responses.

A Your written reports aren't up to scratch.

B What do mean by that?

Response 1: Oh well, it seems you're making a lot of mistakes and we have to keep redoing things and it takes ages to get anything out.

Response 2: I think it's mainly a proof-reading problem. In the report you handed in yesterday there were eight avoidable mistakes in what should have been the final draft.

Response 2 is the more specific and more likely to lead on to a constructive discussion.

Step 3 – Search for a joint solution

Remember the purpose of criticism is to find a solution. Most people will be more committed to solutions which they have found for themselves or have been genuinely involved in formulating. Avoid the temptation of imposing your own remedy – telling the appraisee what the solution is going to be. The instruction: 'I'll tell you what you need to do', is better replaced by the question: 'Now, how do you think we can tackle this?'

Where possible share the responsibility for action. Use the inclusive 'we' when talking about solutions and offer practical support in helping to overcome specific problems.

When you have built a solution, ensure that you give and get commitment to it. Use summarising techniques to focus attention on agreed action and to minimise the scope for ambiguity and misunderstanding. Establish 'do-by' dates for action and/or progress checks as in the following: 'Okay, so are we agreed? I'm going to do .... You're going to look at .... Can we meet on Monday to check on progress?'

Receiving criticism

Apart from being a valuable attribute in its own right, being able to take criticism is essential if we are to criticise others. This is not merely because understanding how to take criticism may give us a useful insight into how the criticised may feel and respond, but also because, as we have seen, when we criticise someone we will often find ourselves criticised back. Responding positively to criticism directed at us is essential if we are to avoid a vicious circle of criticism, resentment and aggression.

There are three steps to taking criticism which mirror those already identified in the process of giving criticism. These steps are:

Step 1. Listen to the critic and repeat back the criticism.
Step 2. Ask the critic to specify the problem.
Step 3. Search for a solution to the problem.

Step 1 – Listen to the critic

Avoid making an immediately negative, emotional, defensive response. Your objective should be to open up communication on what could be an important issue rather than to shut it down without exploring it properly. Don't deny the criticism, defend yourself, justify yourself, argue or evade the issue. Neither should you simply capitulate and go along with the criticism without exploring it properly.

It's useful to repeat back and clarify your understanding of what is being said to you. In repeating back the criticism, try to rephrase it in a less threatening way. Build empathy and accept that there could be room for a better or alternative approach.

The following example shows alternative ways of handling this process. Response 1 which involves a counter-attack might simply lead to a slanging match. Response 2 is more likely to open a constructive discussion.

You're really being unfair.

Response 1: No, I'm not. You're just being too sensitive.

Response 2: I appreciate that you might feel that way. I certainly want to be as reasonable as I can.

Step 2 – Specify (clarify) the problem

Don't jump to conclusions. Ensure you understand exactly what aspect of your behaviour is being criticised, otherwise you may end up talking at cross purposes. By getting the appraisee to specify the problem, you can help to ensure that the discussion focuses on the situation and doesn't become a personal conflict.

The following example combines both the techniques of repeating the criticism and moving on to focus on the specifics.

You say I'm being unfair. Which specific aspects of the approach seem unreasonable to you?

Step 3 – Search for a solution

It's important to adopt a constructive attitude even if the critic's attitude is negative and hostile. This allows you to move on from the problem to an exploration of what can be done about it. Ask for, or offer, a solution. Try something along the line of: 'Okay, if that's the problem, what do you think I should do about it?' or 'Okay, if that's the problem, would it help if I ...?'

Try to engage your critic in the search for a joint solution. Again, the inclusive 'we' is useful to set the right tone. 'Okay, if that's the problem what can we do about it ...?'

Handling aggression

Finally, a word on handling aggression. Criticism, however well delivered, may provoke an aggressive response. This is something that you need to be able to handle skilfully. There is an obvious danger of aggression breeding aggression as it sparks an immediate and emotional response.

Faced with aggression the 'fight or flight' instinct can be triggered with unfortunate consequences. Control your emotions. Respond in a considered manner, choosing your words and tone carefully to produce the outcome which you want. Of course, instinctive reactions are instantaneous while considered rational thought takes a little longer. There's a lot to be said for the old adage of counting to ten before responding to provocation!

14 *Case studies*

This chapter is designed to help you think through some of the issues which may be involved in conducting appraisals with your own staff and developing with them strategies for improving performance. You may see some parallels between the characters who appear in the case studies and the people you have to appraise. Even where such parallels do not exist, you should find these cases useful in developing your skills in diagnosing performance problems and prescribing remedies.

The organisation and the individuals represented in these case studies are entirely fictitious. In real life the stories and relationships would be far more complex. Here they have been simplified for purposes of presentation and to allow you to identify and analyse the main themes.

Case study 1
Jacqui Brown – Editorial Assistant

The organisation

H&C Publishing, is a small publishing company employing about 80 people full time and a varying number of writers, researchers and consultants on a freelance basis. H&C specialises in publishing research reports, books and training aids for the hotel and catering industry. H&C also produces a monthly magazine called *Catering Monthly* which has a trade circulation of 30,000 copies.

Reporting structure

Jacqui Brown is Editorial Assistant – *Catering Monthly*. Jacqui reports to Sarah Davidson who is the Editor of *Catering Monthly* and Jacqui's appraiser. The reporting structure of the editorial team is represented in Figure 14.1.

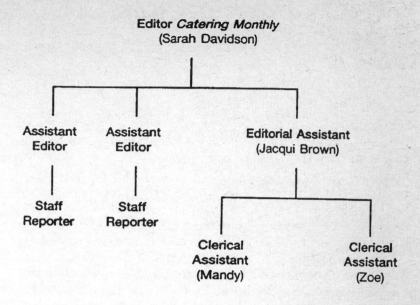

Figure 14.1 *H&C Publishing: editorial team reporting structure – magazines*

The Job

The main purpose of Jacqui's job is to provide an administrative and secretarial support service to the editorial team. A simplified version of Jacqui's job description follows.

Job title: Editorial Assistant
Reporting to: Editor, *Catering Monthly*

Job purpose
To provide administrative and secretarial support to the editorial team.

Main responsibilities
1. Providing a personal secretarial service to the Editor.
2. Coordinating the work of the Clerical Assistants to ensure

---

that the Assistant Editors and Staff Reporters are provided with efficient secretarial support services including: answering the phone, coordinating diaries, filing, maintaining stationery supplies etc.

3. Providing a word processing service to the editorial team and preparing final copy for printing.
4. General administrative duties including monitoring holiday and sick leave and monitoring and recording expenditure of departmental budgets.
5. Keeping the magazine's editorial schedule up to date.
6. Calling the monthly schedule meeting, reporting to it on progress and noting and monitoring agreed action points.

Personal background

Jacqui is 27. She joined H&C 18 months ago to take up her present position working for Sarah Davidson. Jacqui left school at 18 (before completing her 'A' level course) and trained as a secretary. Since then she's held a variety of secretarial and personal assistant posts.

Sarah's perspective

'I'm very happy with Jacqui's overall performance. She is very systematic and efficient. The editorial and publication schedules are always well monitored and maintained. I always receive good personal secretarial service from her. Her typing and word processing are fast and accurate and her knowledge of other computer applications seems good. She is always very willing and personable.

'I have, however, heard some minor grumblings from both the Assistant Editors that they are dissatisfied with the level of secretarial and administrative support they receive. They complain of backlogs and delays in producing word processed copy of articles and have remarked that the work produced by the Clerical Assistants often includes many inaccuracies and has to be resubmitted. They have also complained that filing is not kept up-to-date and that there are frequent instances of misfiling.

'Clearly there is a problem with the Clerical Assistants. Mandy has been in the department for several years. She doesn't seem to be very motivated and is probably happy to do the minimum of work. Zoe has been at H&C only about three months. She came in to replace Jenny, who moved on to take a similar post in another department. Zoe is very young and inexperienced and I don't think she's really found her feet yet. I recruited Zoe, but I consulted with Jacqui about the appointment and she seemed quite happy at the time.'

Jacqui's perspective

'I've been doing this job for about 18 months now. Mostly I enjoy it and get on fairly well with my boss, Sarah. I work very hard. I like to take pride in my work and I'm very efficient at what I do.

'However, I'm not entirely happy with the way the department is run and I don't feel that Sarah really understands my problems. The pressure of work can be tremendous. The Assistant Editors and the Staff Reporters are always making unreasonable demands on my time and resources and this creates problems when it comes to resolving conflicting priorities.

'These problems are made all the worse by Mandy and Zoe.

'Mandy is, quite frankly, lazy. She tries to do as little as possible and needs constant chivvying. She's been in the department several years and knows she has no hope of promotion.

'Zoe, who joined three months ago, is not only very inexperienced but also a bit thick. She's been extremely slow to pick up our procedures, her basic skills are inadequate and she never seems to learn. Appointing Zoe was Sarah's decision – Sarah introduced me to each of the candidates as she did a tour of the office and asked me what I thought of them. Zoe was probably the best of a bad bunch.

'I think Sarah should get rid of Mandy and Zoe and replace them with someone better – H&C probably needs to offer better wages.

'I'm very keen to keep abreast of office technology and I'd like the opportunity of developing and using my computer skills more – not just word processing, but perhaps spreadsheets, databases and stuff like that I don't really know much about.'

The issues

As in many appraisal situations, there is a difference in the perspective of the appraiser and appraisee. In this particular case these differences are slight. Paradoxically, because they are so slight, there is all the more danger that appraiser and appraisee will not recognise the differences. It's quite possible that, even by the end of the discussion, neither Sarah nor Jacqui will have changed their perspective.

In appraising Jacqui, Sarah has to be careful to review Jacqui's job as a whole, recognising strengths but also concentrating on those areas where there is a shortfall in performance. There's plenty of scope for praise, but Sarah must also be analytical, objective and critical. Because Sarah receives good personal service from Jacqui, there is a danger that she might subconsciously filter out Jacqui's shortcomings in performing other aspects of her job. For instance, Sarah might dismiss the Assistant Editors' 'minor grumblings' as not being really important. In other words, Sarah might be caught out by the 'halo' effect. As part of her preparation for the appraisal, Sarah needs to examine the level of service the Assistant Editors actually receive. If she is to tackle Jacqui on this subject she can't rely on vague grumblings and will need facts to back up any criticism and illustrate the problem.

Sarah will need to structure the discussion to ensure that the problem of the service to the rest of the department is addressed and that some action is agreed on how to deal with it. She will have her own ideas as to where the problem lies, but she must be very careful that she also gathers Jacqui's views.

Jacqui's view would be that the department is under-resourced and that Mandy and Zoe are not up to the job. There may be some value in this point of view, but Sarah has to be very careful not to allow this session to be hijacked by a discussion of Mandy's and Zoe's performances. Jacqui may seek to shift the blame on to them, or even onto Sarah as the manager responsible for under-resourcing the department. It's important that Sarah recognises that Jacqui feels the blame lies elsewhere, otherwise she will probably not appreciate the need to shift Jacqui's perspective. Sarah needs to get Jacqui's attention focused on her own responsibilities, especially those of managing Mandy and Zoe.

It's quite possible that Jacqui has never fully appreciated the importance of this aspect of her job, seeing instead her prime role as providing a personal secretarial service to the Editor. After all, Jacqui's job description talks about 'coordinating the work of the Clerical Assistants' rather than managing the Clerical Assistants. Jacqui needs to be helped to see that staff management is a proactive role.

In discussing the Mandy and Zoe issue, Sarah has to be careful not to buy into Jacqui's prejudices. Unfortunately it's all too easy to assimilate uncritically the views of someone like Jacqui, who overall is a good and willing member of staff. Sarah needs to get Jacqui thinking about why Mandy is demotivated and what she could do to motivate her, and why Zoe is poor at picking things up. While Jacqui might push for Mandy and Zoe to be replaced, this (even if possible) is not the answer. Jacqui might manage any replacement staff equally badly. Why, after all, did Jenny leave to go to a similar job on the same grade?

Solutions need to be found in terms of getting Jacqui to create a more motivating job for Mandy, perhaps providing more variety or responsibility or a closer personal working relationship with the Assistant Editors. Quite possibly, Jacqui's management style of 'chivvying' Mandy has been counterproductive. Zoe needs to be given more of Jacqui's attention – at least in the short to medium term. Tasks must be carefully selected so that Zoe can both work within, and gradually expand, her abilities. There is no point in swamping her. Jacqui could benefit from attending a short course on supervisory skills or perhaps on the skills of on-job training . It's not necessarily the case that Zoe's thick: it may be that Jacqui's rather poor at showing her what to do and coaching her in a structured manner.

Other actions might include some initiative to get Assistant Editors to do more forward planning, giving advanced notice and clearer specification of deadlines. This may be an issue for Sarah to take on board at the monthly schedule meeting.

Sarah should also be aware that she might herself be a major part of Jacqui's problem – perhaps she gets good service because her work is given priority at the cost of others. Jacqui may be prioritising on the basis of power (doing jobs for the boss first) without Sarah recognising that this is distorting the priorities of the department as a whole.

Sarah and Jacqui might also usefully review the procedures which led to Zoe's appointment. Perhaps Jacqui needs to be more involved in selecting staff so that she feels greater commitment to the decisions made. Any initiatives to get Jacqui more involved may mean that she would benefit from training in staff selection techniques.

Case study 2
Peter Philips – Assistant Editor (Books)

The organisation

H&C Publishing (see Case Study 1)

Reporting structure

Peter Philips is Assistant Editor – Books. Peter reports to Helen Smith, Editor – Books and Training Aids. Peter has no staff reporting to him.

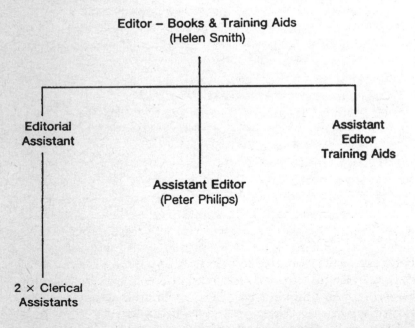

Figure 14.2 *H&C Publishing: editorial team reporting structure – books*

The job

The main purpose of Peter's job is to manage the publication of new books, new editions and reprints through their development from concept to completion. Books are published on a speculative basis – that is to say they are not commissioned by client organisations (as may be the case with some of H&C's research projects). A simplified version of Peter's job description follows.

Job title: Assistant Editor – Books

Reporting to: Editor – Books and Training Aids

Job purpose
To manage the publication of new books, new editions and reprints, throughout their various stages of development from concept to completion.

Main responsibilities
1. To assist the Editor in the formulation of publishing policy by identifying and assessing opportunities for new titles.
2. Commissioning freelance authors to write books and liaising with them thereafter throughout the various stages of production.
3. Copy-editing manuscripts.
4. Proof-reading and passing for final printing.
5. Production management including liaison with designers and selecting and commissioning printers.
6. Agreeing print runs with the Editor.
7. Working in cooperation with the Marketing and Circulation Manager to produce promotional copy and marketing strategy for new books.

Personal background

Peter is 24. He graduated less than three years ago with a good degree in English from a respected university. On graduating he joined a large publishing firm, MacLongs, as an Assistant Editor where he worked in the leisure interest section publishing 'coffee table' books. Peter joined H&C about nine months ago and this will be his first full and formal appraisal. Since joining the department Peter has completed work on five books, which were already in the pipeline at various stages of development. He has also started work on eight new titles which should be published over the next six months.

Helen's perspective

'Peter is bright, very hard working, self-disciplined and shows considerable creative flair. He is also extremely self-confident, perhaps too much so. Since he joined us his output has been prodigious and, on the whole, I'm pleased with the content and design of each of the books produced.

'There have, however, been one or two problems. Although I've mentioned them before, I'll need to discuss them again with Peter. One of his books dealt with kitchen hygiene. The trade press reviews were okay, but we have had a few complaints regarding some of the details such as illustrations showing kitchen staff wearing their hair loose and using wooden chopping boards. Another of Peter's books was *Fire in Hotels*. Unfortunately we got some adverse comment from the fire brigade. They pointed out that while the book dealt with fire hazards and evacuation, it failed to deal adequately with firefighting techniques such as the use of the correct fire extinguishers.

'Another major issue I need to raise is Peter's failure to keep costs within budget. It has now become apparent that each of the titles Peter has so far produced has exceeded the original production cost estimate. We need to keep production costs down (or at least ensure that costs are accurately forecast when investment decisions are made). When a project goes over budget it can easily lose its commercial viability.

'Actually, I think Peter's commercial judgment is a little questionable. He's made a number of suggestions for new titles, but none of them have been worth pursuing. They tended to involve high levels of investment for very uncertain returns.'

Peter's perspective

'This is my first appraisal. I've been in the job for nine months. I'm now on top of things and am looking forward to having an increasingly important impact on publishing policy. I work hard, usually late into the evening and sometimes at weekends. I take a great deal of pride in my work and am ambitious to get on.

'Even if I say it myself, I've got considerable creative flair and originality. Unfortunately, this is not being properly recognised at H&C. When I worked at MacLongs we placed far greater emphasis on content and design and I think high standards in these areas are vitally important. At H&C we seem to place too much emphasis on deadlines – getting the book out quickly – which is often to the detriment of design standards and quality. Design standards really do need improving. During the time I've been here I've completed work on five books with which I'm very pleased. I believe I've set an example of the sort of design improvements H&C could make.

'I know I've been a little over budget on each of the titles I've produced. But this was really due to the pressure of deadlines forcing me to make use of more expensive printing than was originally envisaged (rush jobs cost extra). This really just reinforces my point that the deadlines and budgets we set are too tight if we're to produce quality books. For instance, the criticisms we had over _Kitchen Hygiene_ and _Fire in Hotels_ reflect the fact that deadlines were so tight that there wasn't enough time to circulate final drafts to outside consultants before publication.

'I'm really disappointed that I haven't been given more scope to develop my own publishing policy. At MacLong's I was concerned purely with production. I was attracted to this job because it offered me the opportunity to be more proactive, deciding what should be published and commissioning authors accordingly. In fact, every time I come up with a good idea, Helen seems to reject it out of hand on the grounds that it won't sell. I think she's far too cautious in projecting sales. She needs to be prepared to take more risks in breaking new ground.'

The issues

Peter has a high opinion of himself and needs to be handled carefully. His performance is not as good as he thinks it is and he needs a corrective view. In situations such as these, however, there is a danger the appraisee may totally dominate the discussion, declaring his/her own virtues, criticising the organisation and 'swamping' the appraiser. Helen mustn't let this happen as the appraisal would then be a lost opportunity. However, she must also resist the temptation to attack Peter as she might destroy his confidence or alienate him. Helen will have to be assertive. She must be prepared to listen to Peter and to acknowledge the validity of his views. At the same time she must ensure that she doesn't lose sight of her own agenda and her objective of getting Peter to see things differently.

Many of the main issues here are interrelated and revolve around quality, time management, budgets and commercial realism. Peter is concerned about 'quality' and regards it as the highest good. Helen has to be more pragmatic, considering how to get the best returns on effort and investment. Marginal improvements in quality often require a large investment of time and effort which may be disproportionate to the gains. Helen has to help Peter see that commercial viability is the ultimate criteria against which they need to perform at H&C. Of course, Peter may have some valid points regarding the tightness of budgets and deadlines. Helen needs to listen to these and see what can be done to make things easier. At the same time, she needs to ensure that Peter recognises that the challenge of the job is to produce as high a standard as possible within the constraints of the resources which are available.

Part of the problem may be that Peter is managing his time badly. He may be aiming for perfection and spending too much time on detail at an early stage and so falling behind schedule, then having to cut corners thus leaving insufficient time for consultation and checking. In terms of training needs, Peter may benefit from help in personal organisation in project management. Personal organisation needs might be met by offering Peter a one- or two-day time-management course. Such a course would allow him the scope to take stock of his current working practices and examine ways in which he could enhance his personal efficiency. Project management needs might be met by a series of coaching sessions with Helen in which they plan together the project schedules and critical paths for the next books. Peter also needs help in developing his commercial acumen. Here, a course on finance for the non-financial manager with particular emphasis on investment appraisal might be useful. On the other hand, it might be more worthwhile if Peter spent some time on a short-term secondment to the marketing department to develop his commercial understanding.

There is one very important difference in Helen and Peter's perspectives which hopefully Helen will realise and address during the course of the appraisal discussion. Peter sees his job as being about developing *his own* publishing policy and feels frustrated that he's being held back. Indeed, he says this was the main thing which attracted him to H&C. Helen really sees Peter's job as being to carry out *her* publishing policy, although he's expected to contribute ideas. This confusion may have arisen because of some off-the-cuff remark that Helen might have made at Peter's selection interview, such as 'If you join us you'll be in a position to develop publishing policy.' One of the objectives of appraisal should be to check out if the appraisee's understanding of the job (and what constitutes its important elements) is the same as that of his/her boss. This can be particularly important in the case of an appraisee who has only recently been appointed.

Lastly, Helen has to be very careful about how she raises the issue of the two books about which there have been complaints. She says that she needs to raise this issue with Peter, but Peter has already been made aware of the criticisms. Helen shouldn't go over old ground. She should only raise these issues again if analysing the causes helps her and Peter to develop their understanding of how he could improve in his job. In this instance, they can be used as a basis to explore the issue of the constraints under which Peter has to operate and might provide useful clues to the fundamental factors affecting Peter's performance.

One of the significant lessons to draw from this case study is the need to listen to the appraisee (however difficult he/she may be). While we saw in the previous case study (Sarah and Jacqui) that it was important for the appraiser to change the appraisee's perspective, we should remember that appraisal is also an opportunity for the appraiser to gain new insights and test their own understanding of the situation. In this case Peter sees deadlines as the critical issue. Helen, however, may not be aware of the problem as all of the books have actually been completed on time. Unless Helen engages Peter in the discussion and listens to him, she may miss this fundamental point.

Case Study 3
Brian Hughes – Research Officer

The organisation

H&C Publishing (see Case Study 1)

Reporting structure

Brian Hughes is one of two Research Officers working for Tony Jacobs who is the Editor – Research Reports and Surveys. The other Research Officer is Jayne McCarthy with whom Brian shares a secretary, Sue Williams.

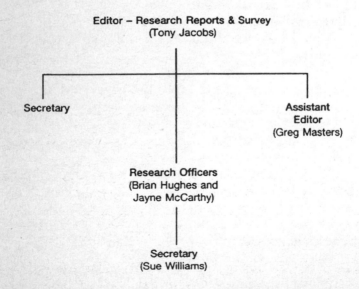

Figure 14.3   *H&C Publishing: research department reporting structure*

The job

The department produces a wide range of research reports for the catering industry, covering topics such as employment trends, developments in vocational education and training, new technology, market trends and so forth. Some of these reports will be produced speculatively (ie where H&C thinks that a subject is important and/or a report will sell well); other reports are commissioned by the government, industry bodies or large firms.

Brian's role is to manage the research stage of chosen projects and to work with the Assistant Editor (Greg Masters) in preparing reports for publication. A simplified version of Brian's job description follows.

Job title: Research Officer

Reporting to: Editor, Research Reports and Surveys

Job purpose
To manage and research projects and prepare reports for publication.

Main responsibilities
1. Proposing to the Editor suitable areas for research projects and surveys and identifying possible clients to commission research.
2. Planning and implementing research projects.
3. Identifying and working with outside specialists on a project by project basis.
4. Designing and applying questionnaires and interpreting statistical data so acquired.
5. Writing up research findings and, in coordination with the Assistant Editor, preparing them for publication.

Personal background

Brian is 51. He's been working for H&C for 15 years, the last 12 of which have been in his current post. Before joining H&C Brian worked in a civil service department and before that spent a couple of years teaching at a polytechnic. Brian has a master's degree in Sociology. Brian didn't go to university until he was 27, until that age he worked in the family's retail furniture business.

Tony is 31. He's only been in his post as Editor – Research Reports and Surveys for the last five months. Tony was appointed from outside H&C. Brian was one of the rejected applicants for the same post.

Tony's perspective

'I'm worried about Brian and his performance. There's an undercurrent of tension between us. Brian did, of course, apply for my job and is probably resentful that he didn't get it.

'Brian's got a good reputation. In the past his work has always been good and over the years he's been responsible for producing some very significant and highly valued reports.

'However, current performance is not up to scratch. He appears stale, lethargic and even cynical. He's no longer putting forward any ideas for new projects and dismisses out of hand proposals put forward by other members of the editorial team. The amount of time he spends out of the office on 'field research' and its associated costs has been rising steadily over the last few months. I'm not accusing him of being on the fiddle, but I am concerned that he's not making the best use of time and resources allocated to him.

'I'm also concerned about his relationships with other members of the team. Greg has complained that Brian's material is usually submitted to him later than he would like and that it's in a format which makes his job more difficult than it need be. I don't think he gets on with Jayne. I've certainly heard them exchange some fairly sarcastic comments. Sue, the secretary Brian shares with Jayne, seems to be pretty poorly briefed and never seems to know where he is.'

Brian's perspective

'I'm really very fed up. I've been with H&C for 15 years and been doing the same job for the last 12. Over that period I've done a good job and produced some really good studies, but I don't get the appreciation or the recognition I deserve.

'I applied for the job as Editor – Research Reports and Surveys last year. With my experience I should have walked into the job, but instead they appointed a 'whiz kid' from outside. I'm very worried about the lack of promotional prospects at H&C. What's the point of doing a good job, if you don't get any rewards in terms of career progress? I've started taking a look around for jobs elsewhere.

'There are other problems as well. I don't really get on with the other members of the department. Jayne's a creep and is always seeking to ingratiate herself with Tony. Greg's also a pain in the neck – always going on about pressure of deadlines and complaining that my copy requires too much subediting. And as for Sue, the secretary I share with Jayne, she's hopeless. She's totally disorganised and expects to be told how to do everything. She's got no sense of priority and often gives preference to non-urgent work for Jayne over work I need doing straight away.

'I've started spending a lot of time out of the office recently working on field research. Quite frankly, I'm pleased to get out and about and away from everyone.'

The issues

This is one of the most difficult situations any manager may have to handle – a relatively young manager responsible for managing an older, experienced person who had applied unsuccessfully for the same job.

For the older employee the experience can be very painful. Failure to get the job perhaps brings home to them that they have reached their career peak and are no longer likely to make any career progress in terms of moving up the organisation's hierarchy. Some people may adjust well to this situation, accepting that they have reached their peak and finding their job satisfaction in factors other than career progression. Others, by contrast, can be thrown into a mid-life crisis and suffer depression, possibly losing their sense of purpose.

Tony has to handle Brian carefully. He's recognised that there's tension between them and that Brian may think he can do the job better than he does. Tony should be criticised for not tackling his problems with Brian sooner. Appraisal is not really the right time to deal with this matter. After a month or two spent establishing himself and then another month or so (subconsciously) avoiding the difficulty, Tony must now face the issue square on. Some managers might be tempted to ignore the problem, arguing that there is really nothing to be done and no benefit in raising the issue and possibly bringing conflict out into the open. It's not uncommon for managers and job-holders to engage in a mutual conspiracy of silence where both parties avoid what they know to be a contentious issue. However, if Tony was to ignore the problem, matters would only get worse. Although he shouldn't have put it off to appraisal, ignoring it now would make a mockery of the appraisal process and probably mean that the issue would never be tackled.

Tony needs to clarify in his own mind what he wants to achieve in his discussion with Brian. He might be tempted to placate him with vague promises of future promotion, but Brian is likely to realise that opportunities are limited and that promotion is unlikely. Tony might be tempted to encourage Brian to look for jobs elsewhere – after all, this would get Brian 'out of his hair'. Both these strategies are flawed as Brian is not likely to be able to move on and Tony will still be faced with managing a demotivated and alienated Brian. Tony's only viable strategy, therefore, must be to remotivate Brian and get the best from him. After all, Brian has a good track record and has previously made a good contribution to the organisation. Tony has a responsibility to ensure that the benefits of Brian's experience and the potential contribution he could make are not lost.

Frankness is called for. Tony needs to voice his concerns, but he also needs to convince Brian that he is a valued member of the organisation. Brian needs to be helped to see that there are other sources of job satisfaction apart from promotion. He also needs to be helped to see that he isn't some sort of inferior being, just because he didn't get promotion. Rather, he may have failed to get promotion simply because he wasn't suited for the managerial role and his talents lie elsewhere.

Tony needs to look at Brian's job design, perhaps giving him more scope for autonomy and opportunities for self-realisation within his work. At the same time, Tony needs to discuss

Brian's relations with his colleagues and work on helping to create a stronger sense of team identity between members of the department.

Brian has his grumbles. They may be the product of his demotivation, but some of his criticisms of colleagues could be well founded. Tony must be wary of the 'horns' effect. Just because Brian is a pain in the neck, doesn't mean that he's wrong about everything! Tony needs to support him and find practical solutions which could take some of the pressure off and help to produce better working relationships all round. Supporting Brain and putting himself out on his behalf is one of the ways Tony can show that he values his contribution.

Case Study 4
Yasmin Khan – Personnel Officer

The organisation

Garden Games Ltd employs some 180 people. It manufactures and markets a range of games for use in the garden. Product lines include: badminton sets; croquet sets; garden chess; bowls; volley ball sets; table tennis sets. GG's target market is the suburban family with a medium-sized garden. GG sells through retail chains, garden centres and by mail order.

A typical games pack will consist of a number of items. For example, the badminton set comprises:

- four rackets;
- one net;
- two net stands;
- one pack of six shuttlecocks;
- one court-liner pack.

The court-liner pack is one of GG's own patented inventions. It consists of rolls of white plastic tape for marking court lines and a packet of pegs for securing the lines in place. GG manufactures its own nets and the patented court-liner packs, but most of the component items for the games sets are bought in from other suppliers. Packing the various components to make up the games sets is therefore a central aspect of GG's operations.

Reporting structure

Yasmin Khan is the Personnel Officer and reports to Ian Cameron who is the Finance and Administration Director. Ian's responsibilities encompass personnel but he is an accountant by profession and Yasmin is the only personnel specialist in the organisation. Yasmin has no staff reporting directly to her but may call upon the support of the clerical assistants in the department (see Figure 14.4).

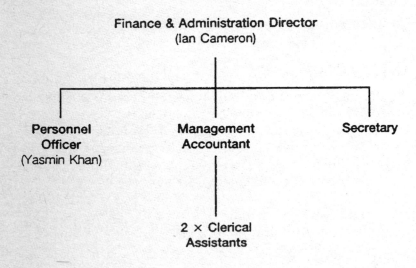

Figure 14.4 *Garden Games Ltd: reporting structure – Personnel Officer*

The job

The purpose of Yasmin's job is to provide a personnel administrative function to the company as a whole. A simplified job description follows.

Job title: Personnel Officer

Reporting to: The Finance and Administration Director

Staff responsibilities: None (but may call upon the resources of the department clerical staff)

Job purpose
To provide a personnel administrative function to the company as a whole.

Main responsibilities
1. Placing job advertisements, sifting and passing on applications to person responsible for post, arranging interviews, formally informing successful and unsuccessful applications.
2. Answering employee queries on payroll, pensions, sickness benefit, holiday entitlement, discipline and grievance procedures, etc.
3. Ensuring that personnel procedures and practices are kept up to date and that the company is aware of the implications of any new legislation on its procedures.
4. Administering the training and conference budget and making arrangements to send people on training courses and conferences.
5. Administering the appraisal system, specifically despatching forms to appraising managers and monitoring their completion.
6. Administering the staff social fund and organising the firm's Christmas and summer functions.

Personal background

Yasmin is 26. She left school after 'A' levels and has since studied for, and attained, her Institute of Personnel and Development qualification. She's been in her current post for the last four years.

Ian's perspective

'Yasmin does a good steady job and is a very valuable member of staff. All her previous appraisals have been very good. She knows her field well and is a source of sound advice. This is essential as I'm not a personnel specialist myself.

'It's a minor criticism, perhaps, but Yasmin can sometimes be a little bit too detailed and technical in the background information she provides. Sometimes I have to wade through more than I really need to know to get to the meat of the argument. Her annual report was very extensive – with its graphs, charts and tables, it was really a bit over the top. I wonder how long it took her to do.

'I'm more concerned about the overspend of the training and conference budget. I know the overspend was caused by the MD and Sales Director deciding late in the year to attend a special conference on exporting after most of the budget had been committed. Nonetheless, I'm keen that we should devise means of planning and controlling expenditure within budgetary disciplines. Of course the money's always tight – the MD considers training, and indeed personnel in general, to be a rather low priority.'

Yasmin's perspective

'I've been in this job for the last four years and I've always done a very competent job. I know my field well and Ian relies on me for good technical advice in personnel matters. I always give very comprehensive and detailed briefs as required. I'm particularly proud of my annual report which I thought was very extensive and, even if I say it myself, very well presented.

'I enjoy my job but don't feel that my talents and professional expertise are being fully utilised. Not being a personnel specialist, Ian has a rather passive and limited idea of what the personnel function should do. I want to develop a far more proactive role.

'A good illustration is the way we manage training. My role is purely administrative, making arrangements on behalf of department heads to send people on specified courses. Occasionally I'm asked to suggest courses to meet a particular need, but my role is largely reactive. The training budget is woefully inadequate and has to cover conference attendance as well. Last year we overshot the budget because the MD and the Sales Director decided they wanted to go on an exporting conference without regard to other spending priorities. I'd like to see training given a higher priority and more resources. I'd like to take a more proactive role developing a training strategy and a personnel development plan for each employee. A lot of what I currently do could be delegated to an administrative assistant leaving me free to take on higher level work. It's very frustrating not having anyone reporting to me to handle administrative detail.

'I like working for Garden Games and family circumstances would make it difficult for me to move to find another job. Nonetheless I want to make career progress and the time is ripe.'

The issues

The main issue here is Yasmin's career aspirations and her desire to create a more proactive role for herself. It's important for the significance of this topic to be identified at the outset of the appraisal discussion. Unless he is aware of it, Ian may waste a lot of time talking about relatively minor matters while Yasmin becomes increasingly frustrated. Even worse, Ian might miss the whole point of Yasmin's concern if, for instance, he flags up that he wants to talk about training budgets and she agrees that she wants to as well. For Ian this issue means tighter budgetary control, for Yasmin it means expanding the budget to fit the new role she has in mind for training.

When we looked at the importance of agendas (see Chapter 11), I emphasised that agenda building should be a joint process. However, simply asking an appraisee what issues they want to talk about may not be good enough – you may need to explore in a little more detail which aspects of the issue they are concerned about before you'll be able to fit it into the agenda. In other words, you should probe sufficiently to ensure that you have a common understanding of what an agenda item means before proceeding. (However, in opening up the conversation in this way there's a danger that you may go into too much detail too early – getting drawn into one particular issue before completing the agenda building phase.)

Presuming that the discussion does focus on Yasmin's career aspirations, Ian needs to be careful in handling the subject and ensure that he doesn't give commitments he will be unable to meet or build up Yasmin's expectations unreasonably. Just because a more proactive role for personnel fits with Yasmin's career aspirations, it doesn't mean to say that Garden Games needs someone to take on the role that Yasmin would like. Even if Ian is sold on Yasmin's ideas, he must caution her about expecting too much. The MD doesn't place a great deal of emphasis on training and personnel and Yasmin needs to be realistic about what may be achieved.

Ian cannot give Yasmin what she wants. The best he can do is to give her the opportunity to prepare and present a case for the changes she wants to make. Even if the argument might be unpopular with the MD, Ian should be prepared to help and coach Yasmin in preparing the best case she can. It may be that Yasmin will have to leave Garden Games if she is to fulfil her aspirations. At least, however, Ian can help her clarify the issue in her own mind and give her every chance to get the MD's support for the role she'd like to take on.

One other minor performance issue in this Case Study is Yasmin's report writing. Her tendency to write reports which are too long and contain irrelevant material is a common failing. People are often tempted to include all the information that they've uncovered rather than selecting only the material necessary to meet the report's objectives. Most readers like short reports and most writers could do with making their reports more reader-friendly. Ian might recommend that Yasmin find a good report writing course. It would need to be one which emphasised structure, relevance and presentation, rather than one which concentrated on punctuation and grammar – aspects which might be more relevant to someone needing help with basic literacy. Training courses can't just be selected on the basis of a generic title, such as 'Report Writing' or even 'Advanced Report Writing' – it's the content and approach that counts.

Case Study 5
Joe Miller – Caretaker/Supervisor

The organisation

Garden Games (see Case Study 4)

The reporting structure

Joe Miller is Garden Games' Caretaker/Supervisor. He reports to Chris Lomax the Maintenance Superintendent. Joe is responsible for five part-time cleaning staff. He also has reporting to him one youth training scheme lad – Steve Mason (see Figure 14.5).

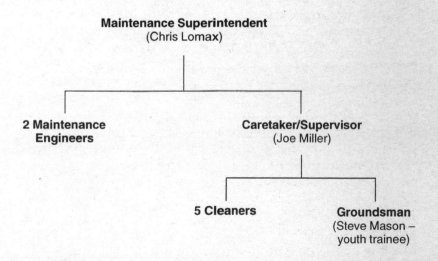

Figure 14.5 _Garden Games Ltd: reporting structure –_
Caretaker/Supervisor

The job

The main purpose of Joe's job is the upkeep and cleanliness of the buildings and grounds.

A simplified version of Joe's job description follows.

Job title: Caretaker/Supervisor

Reporting to: Maintenance Supervisor

Staff responsibilities: 5 part-time cleaners; 1 youth trainee groundsman/handyman

Job purpose
To ensure the upkeep and cleanliness of the buildings and grounds.

Main responsibilities
1. To recruit and supervise cleaning staff.
2. To supervise and develop the youth trainee groundsman/handyman.
3. To carry out small routine repairs and maintenance tasks.
4. To select and supervise outside contractors when specialist maintenance services are required (such as painters, plumbers, electricians).
5. To maintain all gardens and lawns.
6. To maintain all gardening and cleaning equipment.

Personal background

Joe is 48. He's been in his present job for the last seven years. Previously he was a self-employed builder/handyman.

Joe's boss Chris (aged 39), has only been in post for the past eight months. During this period Chris has set out to systemise a lot of the working practices which come under his responsibility.

This is the first time Joe's been appraised as this is the first year Garden Games has extended its appraisal system to cover the sort of grades occupied by Joe.

Chris's perspective

'Joe's not a bad type. He's technically very competent. Certainly the lawns and gardens always look very good. Emergency repairs are always dealt with promptly even if on a makeshift basis.

'But Joe can be a bit "difficult". He always wants to do things his own way and can't see the importance of sticking to procedure.

'I've made some progress with him. When Mavis, one of the cleaners left, Joe wanted to take on Joan, his sister-in-law. I got him to go through a formal recruitment procedure. Joan got the job in the end – not through knowing the right person, but because she was the best of the bunch of applicants. I'm still not sure Joe's convinced that we had to do it that way.

'I'm also rather concerned about Steve, the youth trainee lad who reports to Joe. I've seen him hanging around a fair amount. He complains that he hasn't got anything to do and that the job's "boring". I really need to find out where the problem lies and what can be done about it.

'I also need to get Joe to change the way he hires painters, plumbers and other contractors. I've got to make sure we always get the best deal. I get the feeling Joe tends to give the business to people he likes and has worked with before rather than looking for the best deal.'

Joe's perspective

'I've been doing my job for the last seven years and doing it pretty well. Now they've brought in this appraisal nonsense and I've got to let Chris Lomax interview me to tell me how I'm performing. It's all a waste of time and I can't really see it doing any good.

'Actually it's quite typical of what's going on round here, ever since Chris took over. Now I'm not saying it's his fault and I suppose he's okay really, but him and the senior management have gone systems mad – it's all rules, regulations and procedure now. Look what happened when Mavis left. I'd already got Joan lined up for the job. In the old days I'd have just signed her on, but Chris forced me to go through a boring formal recruitment procedure which was just a waste of time – Joan ended up getting the job just the same. Of course I can see the point when you're recruiting a manager or something, but for a part-time cleaner – I ask you, what next? He's probably going to want to interfere next in the way I hire the painters or the tarmac men – more bloody forms and red tape.

'What I really need is some more help. I told Chris this just after he started, but instead of getting me someone who knew what they were doing, they foisted this lad Steve on me. Chris said they wanted to give a youngster a chance. I reckon they just wanted to save a bit of money. Steve's okay, but because he hasn't got any experience, there are a lot of things he can't do, so he spends quite a bit of time hanging round doing nothing and I'm left doing as much as before.'

The issues

Joe isn't convinced that the new appraisal system is worthwhile, and may even be openly hostile. It's important for Chris to anticipate this difficulty and do his best prior to the appraisal round to 'sell' Joe the benefits of the system, encouraging him to take an active part and to come along well prepared for the appraisal discussion.

Even if he's made some progress towards this, it's still probably useful for Chris to clear the air and get Joe's feelings out in the open at the beginning of the discussion. He might try something like: ' Before we get down to details, I'd just like to talk with you about the appraisal system and your feelings about it.' If Joe's negative attitude comes across, Chris might try to persuade Joe of the benefits of the appraisal process. But he must be careful or this could be counterproductive. Joe may not be for persuading and feel that he's entitled to his own point of view, no matter what Chris says.

Even if he can't persuade Joe of the value of appraisal, Chris mustn't let Joe's cynicism prevail. In other words, Chris has got to maintain his support for the system and not agree with Joe that it's a waste of time.

The same also applies to the issue of the new recruitment procedure which Chris has indicated he wants to raise as one as one of his agenda items. Chris has to be assertive. Even if Joe doesn't like the recruitment procedure, he's got to put up with it and make it work. Recruiting by word of mouth may or may not be inefficient, but it certainly has implications for an equal opportunities employment policy and the legal obligation of the firm to recruit fairly.

Unfortunately, because Chris has to be assertive in respect of the recruitment system, he may find himself at loggerheads with Joe on other issues, particularly that of hiring of contractors. Because Chris has to tell Joe that he _will_ recruit in a particular way, there is a danger that Chris will try to enforce his will with regard to appointing contractors. However, there is scope for give and take and Chris needs to listen to Joe and respect his views. Chris might be tempted to impose a strict tendering system, but there are other ways, such as price testing, and Chris needs to get Joe's help in bringing out such ideas. This is unlikely to happen if Chris forces his views on Joe. The result may be that Joe acquiesces to Chris's policy but still resents and opposes it: 'Oh well, if that's the way he wants it, I'll do what he wants and wait for it to fail.'

Steve is also another important issue. Here the problem lies in Chris's and Joe's different perspectives as to what Joe's relationship should be to Steve. Joe has failed to see that he needs to act not just as a supervisor but also as a trainer. Joe may need help in developing the skills he needs to provide structured on-job training for Steve. Unfortunately, Steve's experience as a trainee is common. Companies may take on young people and then put them to work under supervisors who are not properly trained in the supervisor/trainer role.

Chris is more than partly to blame. Steve isn't an assistant for Joe – he's an extra responsibility. Chris and Joe now have to make the best of a bad situation, but Chris may gain credibility and respect by acknowledging that he was at fault in making the appointment as a means of providing Joe with extra support. Appraisal can rightly be an occasion for managers to apologise to their staff!

Case Study 6
John Hardy – Supervisor: Packaging Workshop

The organisation

Garden Games (see Case Study 4)

Reporting structure

John Hardy is the supervisor of the packaging workshop. He reports to Paul Wright – Packaging and Despatch Manager. John is responsible for a group of 15 packers (see Figure 14.6).

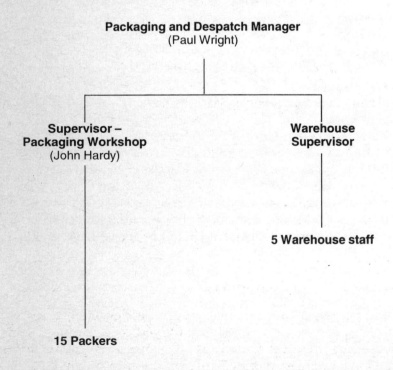

Figure 14.6   *Garden Games Ltd: reporting structure – Supervisor: Packaging Workshop*

The job

The packaging workshop is a central part of Garden Games' operation. Although Garden Games does manufacture some of its own components, most of its operation involves assembling into packs items from diverse sources. Errors (such as putting the wrong net in the volley ball set) are detrimental to Garden Games' reputation for quality and its position in the market. Five years ago GG lost a contract with a major retail outlet because of repeated complaints. GG can't afford for this to happen again. The purpose of John's job is to ensure that quality standards are maintained. John's job description is as follows:

Job title: Supervisor: Packaging Workshop

Reporting to: Packaging and Despatch Manager

Staff responsibilities: 15 packers

Job purpose
To supervise the Packaging Workshop

Main responsibilities
1. To supervise packing staff.
2. To ensure that high standards of quality are maintained. Specifically that:
   - all components and manuals, etc, are packed;
   - all components are packed in the correct way;
   - no obviously faulty components are packed.

Personal background

John Hardy is 31. He's been with Garden Games for six months. He was previously employed as a Foreman Park Keeper by the local council. He was made redundant from that job a year ago and then spent six months on the dole.

Paul Wright is 40. He's held his current position for eight or nine years.

Paul's perspective

'John's doing an okay job considering he's only been with us six months. Of course it's an important job. If it's not done properly we're likely to get customer complaints and returned goods.

'A few months ago, just after John joined, we did have a spell where the number of instances of packaging errors reached an unacceptable level. I had a quiet firm word with John at the time, and impressed upon him the importance of quality. Since then I've not really noticed any problems. I'm quite happy to let John get on with things his own way.'

John's perspective

'I've got my appraisal coming up. I hope I don't get another rollicking. I made a lot of mistakes a few months back and Mr Wright gave me a right talking to – said I was responsible for quality and that we couldn't afford any more mistakes. Well, I do my best, but it ain't easy. I've got to check every one of those packs myself to make sure the packers haven't slipped up. I feel like a policeman and I'm sure the packers think I'm a spy. In fact I think they cock it up on purpose just to see if they can put one over on me.

'It certainly doesn't do any good for my relationship with the packers. They're a difficult bunch to manage. I got on quite well with the lads I had to supervise at the park, but they were cooperative and there were only two of them – this is a totally different ball game.

'Anyway I don't suppose there's much to be done about my problems. All I know is I can't afford to lose this job.'

The issues

There's clearly a difference in perspective between Paul and John. Paul thinks John is doing an 'okay' job, John doesn't think he is. Paul remembers having a quiet firm word with John and regards the incident as something in the past. John remembers the same incident as a 'rollicking' and clearly continues to be very nervous of Paul, hence he adopts a very apprehensive approach to appraisal. John may have prevented a reoccurrence of the batch of errors, but he has done so by taking too much on himself and by adopting a working system which is detrimental to his relationship with the packers and their motivation.

John's very unhappy and he's probably suffering from stress. This is partly a result of his experience of redundancy and unemployment and partly because of the vulnerability he feels in his current job. He feels threatened from above and below.

John needs reassurance and support. The big question is whether Paul is likely to give these to him. Paul is not a good manager. He doesn't really know what's going on – he doesn't even know that John's got problems. Because Paul assumes that everything is okay, the danger is that the appraisal won't uncover the real issues. Certainly Paul cannot rely on John to raise the important points himself as he is somewhat reticent and on the defensive.

As an appraiser, Paul needs to reassure John that appraisal isn't about telling someone off, but about (in part) exploring any problems there might be. He needs to encourage John to talk. John may still not be forthcoming, particularly when it comes to making suggestions for action. While normally appraisers should encourage appraisees to make their own suggestions and solve their own problems, Paul may have to be more proactive and encourage John to contribute with questions and suggestions such as: 'What can I do to help?', 'Would it help if ...?' and so on.

Paul needs to get more involved in John's job – spending more time on the shop floor and seeing the problems for himself. Paul would then be able to have a more meaningful discussion with John about the issues which need to be tackled. These issues might include John's span of control (are 15 packers too many for one person to supervise?), setting measurable standards for quality (what are acceptable standards, what standards are being achieved and what targets can be set for improvement?), systems for quality control and perhaps some supervisory training for John. Such training should address particularly John's need to develop his understanding of group dynamics and team working.

Paul's failure to get involved on the shop floor reminds us

that appraisal can never be a substitute for good day-to-day management and that process known by the acronym MBWA – 'Management By Walking About'.

Checklist 1
Leading an appraisal discussion

Before the meeting

1. Prepare. Gather information. Focus on the relevant issues.
2. Help the appraisee to prepare. Get him/her to think about the issues they want to raise.
3. Choose the right seating arrangement.
4. Ensure that the meeting won't be interrupted.

During the meeting

5. Create a relaxed but positive atmosphere. Use the chat-gap.
6. Recap on the purpose of the meeting to establish a framework and ensure focus.
7. Build an agenda together.
8. Get the appraisee talking early.
9. Let the appraisee put his/her views first – listen carefully and show interest.
10. If the appraisee is reticent or apprehensive, encourage him/her with open questions.
11. Once discussion is under way, steer conversation to the headings identified in the joint agenda.
12. Make sure you cover all key aspects of the job.
13. Praise work well done and be specific in your praise.
14. Point out where you are not satisfied or where you think improvements are needed, but:

    - explain your reasons fully and ensure you can back up your comments with facts;

- work with the appraisee to develop a strategy for making improvements.

15. Avoid over criticising. Ration your criticism and only criticise when doing so can be constructive.
16. Keep the discussion 'partitioned' by dealing with one topic at a time. Don't wander around in an unstructured manner. Use the agenda. Identify action points for each topic – *'who is to do what and by when.'*
17. Summarise from time to time to maintain control and check understanding.
18. At the end, summarise orally all the action points or ask the appraisee to summarise.
19. Try to end on a happy or positive note. Thank the appraisee for his/her participation and contribution.
20. Write up the record of the discussion straight away. Don't leave it a week or more before completing the documentation.

Checklist 2
Taking part in an appraisal discussion: Some guidelines for appraisees

This set of guidelines recognises that the appraisee has an interest in, and a responsibility for, the quality of the appraisal discussion. The appraiser therefore has an important role in helping the appraiser.

1. Prepare for the discussion by reflecting on your own performance, job design, scope for contribution and needs.
2. Help the appraiser produce a relaxed atmosphere. Remember he/she may be feeling nervous too.
3. Respect the 'chat-gap', but don't 'go on' too long. Help the appraiser to 'get down to' the formal business.
4. Agree a framework/agenda for discussion with your appraiser. Identify some of the main areas for discussion.
5. Keep the discussion focused. Avoid straying too far from the subject in hand. Keep track of tangents so that you can return to the main path of the conversation. Use summarising techniques to help you refocus the discussion: *'Can we get back to the point we were discussing?'*; *'We were talking about ...'.*(Note: some tangential discussion is natural and useful, but never lose sight of the structure of the discussion.)
6. Help the appraiser to agree specific action. Encourage him/her to be specific about who is to do what by when. Avoid leaving issues 'in the air' without a specific agreement on action unless it is explicitly agreed that no action is needed or possible. Try to get action agreed before allowing the conversation to move on to another agenda item.

7. Make your own notes on actions/commitments agreed by both parties.
8. Ask the appraiser to explain or elaborate on anything which isn't clear. Check your understanding by summarising.
9. Listen. Don't interrupt. If necessary, gently remind the appraiser that he/she should also let you finish your comments.
10. Respond calmly and positively rather than emotionally to criticism, even if the criticism is inept or unjustified. Focus on building solutions. Ask the appraiser's advice in formulating solutions.
11. Flag up or make a personal note of any additional items that you recognise or remember during the appraisal that you would like to discuss. If, at the end, the appraiser fails to check that you have additional items (*'Is there anything else you'd like to discuss?'*), interrupt to prevent him/her getting into 'closing mode' before your additional items are introduced.

Appendix
Implementing an appraisal system

In Chapter 3, I emphasised that effective appraisal requires committed appraisers and appraisees. Their active involvement is therefore essential in designing or reforming any system. System design also requires a great deal of attention to detail. The following steps are suggestions for any personnel specialist or general manager taking responsibility for implementing a scheme.

1. Draft

Having identified the objectives the organisation wishes to achieve from having an appraisal scheme, draft a set of guidelines to act as a consultation document. A flow diagram showing the stages of the proposed scheme will also be useful.

2. Consult

- Using the draft system, first check with the senior management team that your proposals meet (at least broadly) with their requirements. There's no point in proceeding further if you haven't got their approval.
- Set up a 'focus group' or working party of appraisees and appraisers. These should be a cross section of potential users who will be involved at the sharp end. Their views on the practicality and imperfections of the scheme can be extremely important. This focus group is not intended to be part of a democratic or consensus building exercise. Participants do not have to be elected representatives.

Choose people whose perspective is valid and whose contribution may be constructive. Don't make the mistake of packing the group with 'yes' people. It's always useful to hear what opponents have to say. Those who've been involved in the focus group will (if they feel they've been listened to) have a stake in the system's success and may act as champions for it as their various levels throughout the organisation.

Facilitating the focus group meeting requires skill. It is important that members are given the opportunity to develop their understanding of appraisal so that their comments on the draft system will be well informed. It can make sense to use an outside consultant to manage this process.

- Engage an outside consultant to have a look at your proposed design. From a wider perspective he/she may be able to see problems and pitfalls which you haven't anticipated.

3. Refine

Having consulted, you need to refine your design to incorporate the feedback you've received. It's also worth testing the documentation out by doing a dummy run. Actually completing the documentation (if only for a fictitious appraisee) can be a useful way of identifying some of the shortcomings of form design.

Finalise all support documentation and guidelines. Try to write these in a reader-friendly rather than a bureaucratic style.

4. Agree

You now need to get the formal agreement of the senior management team. By this stage you should also have a detailed timetable for implementation.

5. Inform and Brief

Once senior management has decided to go ahead, it's important that all staff are informed and briefed immediately. Delay may lead to unhelpful rumours via the grapevine.

Choose a briefing system which is appropriate to your organisation's mechanisms and culture. Although you might like to circulate a memo, it's unlikely to be sufficient by itself.

Ensure that everyone knows who they are going to be appraising and who they are going to be appraised by. Also, make sure everyone is aware of the timetable.

6. Train

Specific training, in operating the scheme, identifying training needs, objective setting, and above all leading the appraisal discussion, should be arranged for all appraisers. This may involve a one- or two-day training course. It's best to plan training for groups of 9–12 at a time.

Training, particularly in taking part in the discussion, will also be useful for appraisees. A half-day session might suffice and it may be possible to run these sessions for slightly larger numbers of people at a time.

7. Execute and monitor

Implement the system and monitor its progress. Check on levels of compliance and find out how well appraisals are being conducted.

8. Review

Review and refine the system. Be prepared to make adaptations in the light of experience. Make it clear in your initial design that you expect to make adaptations after the first round.

THE LEARNING CENTRE
HAMMERSMITH AND WEST
LONDON COLLEGE
GLIDDON ROAD
LONDON W14 9BL
0181 741 1688